T0201239

Immunophenotyping for Haematologists

Immunophenotyping for Haematologists

Principles and Practice

Barbara J. Bain, MB BS, FRACP, FRCPath
Professor of Diagnostic Haematology
St Mary's Hospital Campus, Imperial College London
and Honorary Consultant Haematologist
St Mary's Hospital, London, UK

Mike Leach, MB ChB, FRCP, FRCPath
Consultant Haematologist and Honorary Senior Lecturer
Haematology Laboratories and West of Scotland Cancer Centre
Gartnavel General Hospital, Glasgow, UK

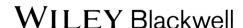

Registered Office(s)
John Wiley & Sons, Inc., 111 River Street, Hoboken, NJ 07030, USA
John Wiley & Sons Ltd, The Atrium, Southern Gate, Chichester, West Sussex, PO19 8SQ, UK

Editorial Office
9600 Garsington Road, Oxford, OX4 2DQ, UK

For details of our global editorial offices, customer services, and more information about Wiley products visit us at www.wiley.com.

Wiley also publishes its books in a variety of electronic formats and by print-on-demand. Some content that appears in standard print versions of this book may not be available in other formats.

Library of Congress Cataloging-in-Publication Data
Names: Bain, Barbara J., author. | Leach, Mike, (Haematologist),
    author.
Title: Immunophenotyping for haematologists : principles and practice /
    Barbara J. Bain, Mike Leach.
Other titles: Immunophenotyping for hematologists
Description: Hoboken, NJ : Wiley-Blackwell, 2020. | Includes
    bibliographical references and index.
Identifiers: LCCN 2020021078 (print) | LCCN 2020021079 (ebook) | ISBN
    9781119606116 (hardback) | ISBN 9781119606147 (adobe pdf) | ISBN
    9781119606154 (epub)
Subjects: MESH: Immunophenotyping | Hematologic Tests
Classification: LCC QR187.I486 (print) | LCC QR187.I486 (ebook) | NLM QW
    525.5.I36 | DDC 616.07/582–dc23
LC record available at https://lccn.loc.gov/2020021078
LC ebook record available at https://lccn.loc.gov/2020021079

Cover Design: Wiley
Cover Images: (background) © KTSDESIGN/SCIENCE PHOTO LIBRARY/ Getty Images,
(inset) courtesy of Mike Leach

Set in 9.5/12.5pt STIXTwoText by SPi Global, Pondicherry, India
Printed and bound in Singapore by Markono Print Media Pte Ltd

10 9 8 7 6 5 4 3 2 1

Contents

Preface

The increasing centralisation of specialised tests and the divorce of clinical from laboratory haematology in many countries means that many haematologists now have no direct contact with an immunophenotyping laboratory. Despite this, the results from the laboratory are often crucial in the management of their patients. This book is intended to help haematologists and trainees understand and interpret immunophenotyping results. It is not directed at those working in an immunophenotyping laboratory and technical details are therefore outlined only briefly. Such laboratories may, however, find it a useful source of information. For further reading on the subject, see the bibliography of each chapter.

Barbara J. Bain and Mike Leach

Acknowledgement

We should like to thank Allyson Doig, Senior Biomedical Scientist, Gartnavel Hospital, for assistance with the flow cytometry plots in Part 4.

Abbreviations Used in the Book

κ	kappa (light chain)
λ	lambda (light chain)
ALCL	anaplastic large cell lymphoma
ALL	acute lymphoblastic leukaemia
AML	acute myeloid leukaemia
AMoL	acute monoblastic/monocytic leukaemia
APC	allophycocyanine
APL	acute promyelocytic leukaemia
AST	aspartate transaminase
ATLL	adult T-cell leukaemia lymphoma
c	cytoplasmic
CAR T cells	chimaeric antigen receptor T cells
CD	cluster of differentiation
CLL	chronic lymphocytic leukaemia
CML	chronic myeloid leukaemia
CMML	chronic myelomonocytic leukaemia
CSF	cerebrospinal fluid
CT	computed tomography
DLBCL	diffuse large B-cell lymphoma
DNA	deoxyribonucleic acid
EBNA	Epstein–Barr virus nuclear antigen
EBV	Epstein–Barr virus
EMA	epithelial membrane antigen
ETP-ALL	early T-cell precursor acute lymphoblastic leukaemia
FBC	full blood count
FISH	fluorescence *in situ* hybridisation
FITC	fluorescein isothiocyanate
FLAER	fluorescent aerolysin
FSC	forward scatter (of light)
G-CSF	granulocyte colony-stimulating factor
GPI	glycosylphosphatidylinositol
Hb	haemoglobin concentration
HHV	human herpesvirus
HIV	human immunodeficiency virus
HLA	human leucocyte antigen
HLH	haemophagocytic lymphohistiocytosis
HTLV-1	human lymphotropic virus 1
Ig	immunoglobulin
IL	interleukin
LDH	lactate dehydrogenase
LGLL	large granular lymphocytic leukaemia
LMP	latent membrane protein
LL	lymphoblastic lymphoma
MALT	mucosa-associated lymphoid tissue
MDS	myelodysplastic syndrome
MDS/MPN	myelodysplastic/myeloproliferative neoplasm
MoAb	monoclonal antibody
MPAL	mixed phenotype acute leukaemia
MPN	myeloproliferative neoplasm
MPO	myeloperoxidase
MRD	minimal residual disease
NHL	non-Hodgkin lymphoma
NK	natural killer
NR	normal range

PE	phycoerythrin	SSC	side or sideways scatter (of light)
PerCP	peridinin chlorophyll	TCR	T-cell receptor
PLL	prolymphocytic leukaemia	TdT	terminal deoxynucleotidyl
PNH	paroxysmal nocturnal		transferase
	haemoglobinuria	ULN	upper limit of normal
RNA	ribonucleic acid	WBC	white blood cell count
Sm	surface membrane	WHO	World Health Organization

Part 1

Purpose and Principles of Immunophenotyping

CONTENTS

Immunophenotyping is the process by which the pattern of expression of antigens by a population of cells is determined. The presence of a specific antigen is recognised by its binding to a labelled antibody. Antibodies can be present in a polyclonal antiserum that is raised in an animal but more often they are well characterised monoclonal antibodies produced by hybridoma technology; a hybridoma is a clone of cells created by the fusion of an antibody-producing cell with a mouse myeloma cell. Monoclonal antibodies can be labelled with an enzyme or with a chemical, known as a fluorochrome, that under certain circumstances will fluoresce. Immunophenotyping is carried out primarily by flow cytometry or immunohistochemistry. Flow cytometric immunophenotyping is applicable to cells in peripheral blood, bone marrow, body fluids (pleural, pericardial, ascitic and cerebrospinal fluids) and fine needle aspirates. Immunohistochemistry of relevance to haematological disease is applied particularly to trephine biopsy and lymph node biopsy specimens, but also to biopsy specimens from any other tissues where infiltration by haemopoietic or lymphoid cells is suspected.

Flow Cytometric Immunophenotyping

This technique determines cell size, structure (to some extent) and antigen expression. Cells in suspension are first exposed to a combination of fluorochrome-labelled monoclonal antibodies (or other lectins or ligands) and then pass in a focused stream through a beam of light generated by a laser. Laser-generated light is coherent (waves of light are parallel) and monochromatic (single wave length/colour). Large multichannel instruments with multiple lasers are used to identify, count, size and otherwise characterise cells that are hydrodynamically focused and pass in a single file through a narrow orifice in a flow cell. The passing of the cell through a light beam leads to both the scattering of light and the excitation of fluorochromes so that they emit a fluorescence signal. Forward

Immunophenotyping for Haematologists: Principles and Practice, First Edition. Barbara J. Bain and Mike Leach.
© 2021 John Wiley & Sons Ltd. Published 2021 by John Wiley & Sons Ltd.

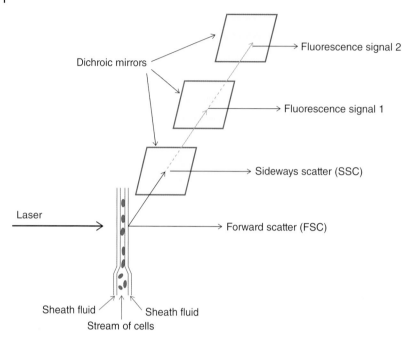

Figure 1.1 Diagrammatic representation of the principles of flow cytometric immunophenotyping.

scatter (FSC) of light at a narrow angle is detected and measured and is proportional to cell size. Sideways or side scatter (SSC) of light is detected and measured and is proportional to cell granularity and complexity. Antigens expressed on the surface membrane of cells or, with modified techniques, within cells are detected. After 'permeabilisation', both cytoplasmic and nuclear antigens can be detected.

For each fluorochrome, a selected laser emits light of a specified wavelength that will be absorbed by the fluorochrome. This leads to excitation of the fluorochrome with subsequent emission of light of lower energy and a longer wavelength as the fluorochrome returns to its basal state; this property is known as fluorescence. The amount of light emitted (the number of photons) is proportional to the amount of fluorochrome bound to the cell. The mean fluorescence intensity of a population indicates the strength of expression of the relevant antigen. The emitted light passes through dichroic mirrors, that is, mir-

rors that reflect some wavelengths and transmit others, so that it is possible, for example, to reflect SSC for measurement and transmit fluorescence signals to another detector such as a photomultiplier tube (Figure 1.1). The detector produces an electrical signal that is proportional to the amount of incident light. Some commonly used fluorochromes are shown in Table 1.1.

The cells that are studied must be dispersed. For peripheral blood and bone marrow aspirate specimens, it is necessary to exclude mature and immature red cells. This is most simply done by lysing red cells using an ammonium chloride solution. Otherwise red cells and their precursors will appear in scatter plots and interfere with gating leucocyte populations of interest. If assessment of immunoglobulin expression is required, there must also be a washing step to remove the plasma that contains immunoglobulin, which would neutralise the monoclonal lambda- or kappa-specific antibody.

Table 1.1   Commonly used fluorochromes.

Fluorescein isothiocyanate (FITC)
Phycoerythrin (PE)
Allophycocyanine (APC)
Peridinin chlorophyll (PerCP)
Cyanine 5 (Cy5), cyanine 5.5 (Cy5.5) and cyanine 7 (Cy7)
Texas red
Pacific blue
Brilliant violet
Krome orange
Alexa Fluor 488 (AF488)
Alexa Fluor 647 (AF647)
Phycoerythrin-Texas Red X (ECD)
Phycoerythrin-cyanine 5 (PE-Cy5)
Phycoerythrin-cyanine 5.5 (PE-Cy5.5)
Phycoerythrin-cyanine 7 (PE-Cy7)

The great majority of monoclonal antibodies used in immunophenotyping have been characterised at a series of international workshops and those with the same specificity have been assigned a cluster of differentiation (CD) number. This number can be used to refer to both the antibody and the antigen it recognises. There are now more than 350 specificities recognised so that a careful selection of antibodies for diagnostic use is important. In addition to fluorochromes conjugated to monoclonal or polyclonal antibodies, it is also possible to use either fluorochromes that can bind directly to cellular constituents, such as DNA, or labelled modified aerolysins that bind to membrane glycosylphosphatidylinositol glycan A (GPI) (used in the diagnosis of paroxysmal nocturnal haemoglobinuria). Propidium iodide binding can be used to identify non-viable cells and exclude them from analysis. Monoclonal antibodies that are most used in flow cytometric immunophenotyping are detailed in Part 2.

Results of immunophenotyping are usually shown as a two-dimensional plot in which FSC, SSC and the expression of certain antigens are plotted against each other, permitting the recognition of the probable nature of a cell cluster in a particular position. It is thus possible to gate on a cellular population of interest. A gate is an electronic boundary; it can either be predetermined or drawn by the operator. There are four commonly used approaches to gating of target populations: FSC versus SSC, CD45 versus SSC, CD19 versus SSC and CD34 versus SSC.

FSC versus SSC is a useful way of screening a specimen to identify normal populations and to highlight abnormal cells as illustrated in Figure 1.2.

Forward scatter is increased in relation to increasing cell size whilst SSC is influenced by cytoplasmic granularity and nuclear complexity. It is a useful means of gating on blasts when CD34 is not expressed, for example in monoblastic leukaemias. Such plots are helpful in identifying large activated lymphocytes, an excess of small lymphocytes or monocytes and even the presence of hairy cells (see Chapter 3). Granular blasts show increased SSC and this is reflected in a shift to the right in the scatter plot. This can be an early indication of a possible acute promyelocytic leukaemia.

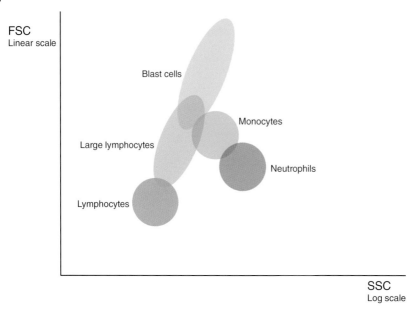

Figure 1.2 Delineation of peripheral blood leucocyte populations using forward scatter (FSC) and side scatter (SSC) characteristics.

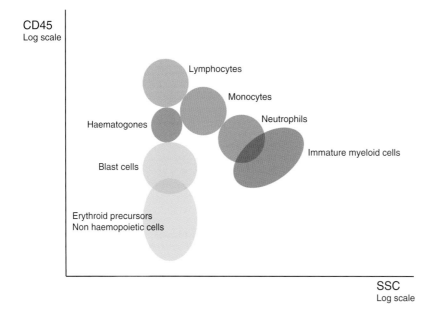

Figure 1.3 Delineation of peripheral blood or bone marrow leucocyte populations using CD45 expression and SSC.

A plot of CD45 expression and SSC is not only useful for separating normal cell populations but also helps identify precursor cell populations, which frequently show only weak CD45 expression (Figure 1.3).

CD19 versus SSC (Figure 1.4) and CD34 versus SSC (Figure 1.5) plots are useful for isolating B cells and blast cells, respectively.

Back gating is a process whereby a target population identified in one approach can be

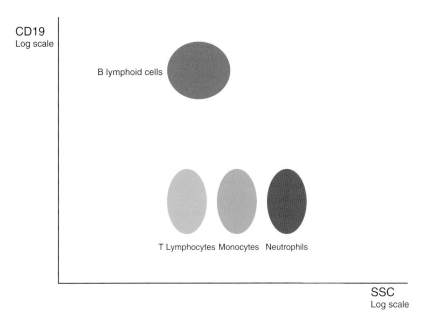

Figure 1.4 Delineation of peripheral blood or bone marrow B-cell populations using CD19 expression and SSC.

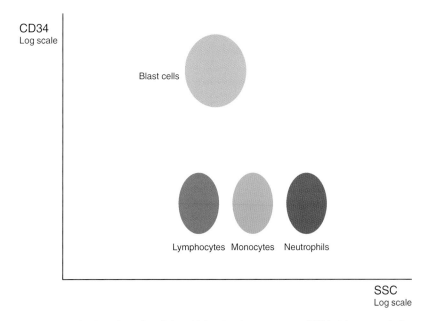

Figure 1.5 Delineation of peripheral blood or bone marrow CD34+ blast populations using CD34 expression and SSC.

tracked in another. For example, CD34+ myeloblasts can be isolated using CD34 versus SSC, then colour tracked into the FSC versus SSC plot to show cell size and granularity. With modern multichannel instruments it is possible to study 6–8 or more antigens in a single tube. If multiple tubes are studied, several core antibody-fluorochrome conjugates can be included in each tube analysed so that cross-comparison between the same cells stained with different antibody panels in different tubes is possible.

Flow cytometric immunophenotyping is used particularly in the investigation of haematological neoplasms, but there are other roles (Table 1.2).

Following analysis, the immunophenotyping laboratory will issue a report detailing the characteristics of any abnormal population identified and offering an interpretation. The

Table 1.2 Role of flow cytometric immunophenotyping.

Haematological neoplasms

Diagnosis of haematological neoplasms

Further classification, e.g. of AML, B-ALL, T-ALL

Identification of disease spread, e.g. to the central nervous system

Identification of a therapeutic target, e.g. CD19, CD20, CD30, CD33, CD52

Detection of minimal residual disease (which may include identifying a leukaemia-specific phenotype at diagnosis)

Identification of hypodiploidy and hyperdiploidy in B-ALL, including the detection of masked hypodiploidy when there has been duplication of a small hypodiploid clone

Investigation of erythrocytes and their disorders

Diagnosis of paroxysmal nocturnal haemoglobinuria (CD15, CD16, CD24, CD55, CD59, CD66b, CD157, FLAER on neutrophils; CD14, CD55, CD157 and FLAER on monocytes; CD55, CD59 and FLAER on erythrocytes) (reviewed in [1])

Identification of a PNH clone in aplastic anaemia (predictive of better prognosis and a response to immunosuppressive therapy)

Diagnosis of hereditary spherocytosis (eosin-5-maleimide binding). Binding is also reduced in hereditary pyropoikilocytosis, South-East Asian ovalocytosis and congenital dyserythropoietic anaemia, type II

Diagnosis of hereditary stomatocytosis due to *RHAG* mutation (reduced expression of CD47, which is part of the Rh protein complex)

Detection and enumeration of fetal red cells in maternal circulation (using anti-RhD when mother is RhD-positive, or using permeabilised erythrocytes and an antibody to haemoglobin F) or using the two techniques in combination

Investigation of platelets and their disorders

Diagnosis of inherited platelet disorders: Glanzmann's thrombasthenia, deficiency of platelet glycoprotein IIb/IIIa (CD41/CD61 absent or reduced in three quarters of patients); Bernard–Soulier syndrome, deficiency of glycoprotein I/V/IX (CD41 and CD42a/CD42b moderately reduced); Scott syndrome (annexin V not expressed on activated platelets); *GFI1B* mutation (CD34 expressed on platelets); Wiskott–Aldrich syndrome (deficiency of WAS protein, reduced or defective CD43 on T lymphocytes)

Investigation of leucocytes and their disorders including investigation of immune function

Investigation of suspected primary immunodeficiency syndromes (reviewed in [2])

Diagnosis of autoimmune lymphoproliferative syndrome (CD3+TCRαβ+CD4−CD8− lymphocytes)

Diagnosis of leucocyte adhesion deficiencies type I (CD18 and CD11a, 11b and 11c deficient) and type II (CD15s deficient); reduced expression of CD11b, CD18 or CD15s by phorbol esterase-stimulated neutrophils is demonstrated

Diagnosis of neutrophil specific granule deficiency (reduced SSC, CD15, CD16, CD66, myeloperoxidase and lactoferrin)

Table 1.2 (Continued)

Diagnosis of chronic granulomatous disease using dihydrorhodamine as a marker of H_2O_2 production after stimulation of neutrophils; carrier detection is also possible

Enumeration of CD4-positive T cells in HIV infection

Investigation for lymphocytic variant of hypereosinophilic syndrome (aberrant phenotypes such as CD3– CD4+CD8– or CD3+CD4–CD8–)

Diagnosis of haemophagocytic lymphohistiocytosis (HLH) (upregulation of HLA-DR on T cells; CD57 and perforin can also be upregulated; testing for deficiency of perforin, SAP, XIAP or CD107a is used to screen for various underlying genetic defects [3, 4]

Diagnosis of persistent polyclonal lymphocytosis

Identification of hypersensitivity by upregulation of CD63 and CD300a on exposure of basophils to a specific allergen [5]

Identification of sepsis by CD64 expression on neutrophils

Other

Enumeration and isolation of haemopoietic stem cells ($CD45^{weak}$, CD34+, SSC^{low})

Differential leucocyte counting; the Beckman Coulter Hematoflow, for example, can distinguish neutrophils, eosinophils, basophils, CD16– and CD16+ monocytes, B cells, CD16+ cytotoxic T cells and NK cells, CD16– T cells, myeloblasts, monoblasts, B lymphoblasts and T lymphoblasts*

Enumeration and characterisation of reticulocytes or platelets by the binding of a fluorochrome (e.g. a proprietary mixture of polymethine and oxazine in Sysmex instruments) to RNA or the binding of a fluorescence-labelled CD61 monoclonal antibody to platelets (CellDyn instruments)*

AML, acute myeloid leukaemia; B-ALL, B-lineage acute lymphoblastic leukaemia; CD, cluster of differentiation; FLAER, fluorescent aerolysin; HIV, human immunodeficiency virus; HLA-DR, human leucocyte antigen-DR; PNH, paroxysmal nocturnal haemoglobinuria; RNA, ribonucleic acid; SAP, SLAM-associated protein; T-ALL, T-lineage acute lymphoblastic leukaemia; XIAP, X-linked inhibitor of apoptosis
* This is not part of conventional immunophenotyping but represents a flow cytometric immunophenotyping technique incorporated into an automated instrument for performing blood counts.

strength of expression of any antigen is also of relevance. This may be expressed as

 i) –, ±, +, ++;
 ii) negative, weak, moderate, strong;
 iii) negative, dim, moderate, bright;
 iv) hi, lo.

It should be noted that ± indicates weak expression whereas +/– indicates that expression may be positive or negative.

An immunophenotyping result will often also be subsequently incorporated into an integrated report that includes the results of other types of investigation, for example, morphological assessment and cell counts, and cytogenetic or molecular genetic analysis.

Immunohistochemistry

Immunohistochemistry predominantly employs a primary monoclonal antibody directed at the target antigen, followed by a secondary anti-immunoglobulin antibody that is coupled to an enzyme; the enzyme can subsequently participate in an enzymatic reaction, producing a coloured product that can be visualised. The most frequently used technique is an immunoperoxidase reaction. For some purposes, for example, the detection of immunoglobulin components, polyclonal antisera may be preferred. Immunohistochemistry has an advantage over flow cytometry in that antigen expression can be related to cytological and histological features. Co-expression of antigens can be studied by using two different enzymatic reactions (such as peroxidase and alkaline phosphatase) or by identifying the same cell population in serial sections of the tissue.

Interpretation and Limitations of Flow Cytometric Immunophenotyping

Flow cytometry must not be interpreted in isolation but in the light of the clinical history, findings on physical examination and the results of other investigations. In particular, the blood or bone marrow film should be carefully examined in the light of the clinical and laboratory findings. Specimens are frequently sent for flow studies where the referring clinician does not have a working diagnosis. For example, a patient presenting with pancytopenia could have a number of potential diagnoses including acute leukaemia, myelodysplastic syndrome, a lymphoproliferative disorder or aplastic anaemia. A morphological review is essential in order that an appropriate panel of antibodies is utilised. Not uncommonly an abnormal cell population in the blood is present at low levels, examples being acute leukaemia, high grade lymphoma and hairy cell leukaemia. The cells identified as being of potential interest morphologically must be correlated with abnormal populations seen in scatter plots so that an appropriate gating strategy is utilised.

Problems and Pitfalls

Clearly technical errors can lead to erroneous results of immunophenotyping. Rigorous quality control is required. Inappropriate selection of antibodies and erroneous interpretation can result from inadequate clinical information being provided or from failure to examine a film of the peripheral blood or bone marrow aspirate that is to be tested. Delays in transportation of a sample to the laboratory can lead to cell death and make testing of the sample unwise since results are likely to be misleading.

Errors in interpretation can occur if the results of immunophenotyping are not integrated with clinical, haematological, cytogenetic and genetic information. Not all cases of a specific condition will have a typical immunophenotype and, in some entities, the immunophenotype is not distinctive.

In certain circumstances flow cytometry of a bone marrow aspirate will show no abnormality despite a neoplastic infiltrate being present. This is likely to occur when there is diffuse or focal bone marrow fibrosis, when the aspirate is of low cellularity and when neoplastic cells are infrequent, fragile or dead. Findings are typically negative in Hodgkin lymphoma where the disease cells, Hodgkin and Reed–Sternberg cells, are present at a low frequency amongst a reactive environment of lymphocytes, plasma cells and eosinophils with associated reticulin fibrosis. In these circumstances it is trephine biopsy histology and immunohistochemistry that yield the diagnosis. It is therefore important not to exclude a diagnosis completely based solely on the results from one approach, particularly where the specimen quality is poor. No single investigation in isolation is infallible – by correlating the results of several investigations using different modalities, a unifying diagnosis can be achieved.

References

1 Illingworth AJ, Marinov I and Sutherland DR (2019) Sensitive and accurate identification of PNH clones based on ICSS/ESCCA PNH Consensus Guidelines. *Int J Lab Haematol*, **41**, Suppl. S1, 73–81.

2 Knight V (2019) The utility of flow cytometry for the diagnosis of primary immunodeficiencies. *Int J Lab Haematol*, **41**, Suppl. S1, 63–72.

3 Ammann S, Lehmberg K, Zur Stadt U, Janka G, Rensing-Ehl A, Klemann C *et al.* for HLH study of the GPOH (2017) Primary and secondary hemophagocytic lymphohistiocytosis have different patterns of T-cell activation, differentiation and repertoire. *Eur J Immunol*, **47**, 364–373.

4 Marsh RA and Haddad E (2018) How I treat primary haemophagocytic lymphohistiocytosis. *Brit J Haematol*, **182**, 185–199.

5 Sabato V, Verweij MM, Bridts CH, Levi-Schaffer F, Gibbs BF, De Clerck LS *et al.* (2012) CD300a is expressed on human basophils and seems to inhibit IgE/FcεRI-dependent anaphylactic degranulation. *Cytometry B Clin Cytom*, **82**, 132–138.

Bibliography

Béné MC (2019) The wonderful story of monoclonal antibodies. *Int J Lab Hematol*, **41**, Suppl. S1, 8–14.

Gorczyca W (2017). *Flow Cytometry in Neoplastic Hematology: Morphologic-Immunophenotypic Correlation*, 3rd edn. CRC Press, Boca Raton.

Leach M, Drummond M and Doig A (2013) *Practical Flow Cytometry in Haematology Diagnosis*. Wiley-Blackwell, Oxford.

Ortolani C (2011) *Flow Cytometry in Haematological Malignancies*. Wiley-Blackwell, Oxford.

Porwit A and Béné MC (2018) *Multiparameter Flow Cytometry in the Diagnosis of Hematologic Malignancies*. Cambridge University Press, Cambridge.

Swerdlow SH, Campo E, Harris NL, Jaffe ES, Pileri S, Stein H and Thiele J (eds) (2017) *WHO Classification of Tumours of Haematopoietic and Lymphoid Tissues, revised 4th edn*. IARC Press, Lyon, pp. 37–38.

Part 2

Immunophenotyping for Haematologists

A Compendium of Antibodies and Patterns of Expression of Equivalent Antigens in Normal and Neoplastic Cells

For more detail on expression of antigens in specific haematological neoplasms, see the bibliography and Part 3 of this book. Cluster of differentiation (CD) numbers describe both the antigen and relevant antibodies. The most commonly used and important antibodies for flow cytometry are highlighted by being in bold.

Abbreviations

ALCL, anaplastic large cell lymphoma; ALL, acute lymphoblastic leukaemia; AML, acute myeloid leukaemia; ATLL, adult T-cell leukaemia/lymphoma; CAR T cell, chimaeric antigen receptor T cell; CLL, chronic lymphocytic leukaemia; CML, chronic myeloid leukaemia; CMML, chronic myelomonocytic leukaemia; DLBCL, diffuse large B-cell lymphoma; EBV, Epstein–Barr virus; G-CSF, granulocyte colony-stimulating factor; GPI, glycosylphosphatidylinositol; HHV, human herpesvirus; HIV, human immunodeficiency virus; HLA, human leucocyte antigen; HLH, haemophagocytic lymphohistiocytosis; HTLV-1, human T-cell lymphotropic virus 1; Ig, immunoglobulin; IL, interleukin; LL, lymphoblastic lymphoma, MALT, mucosa-associated lymphoid tissues; MDS, myelodysplastic syndrome; MDS/MPN, myelodysplastic/myeloproliferative neoplasm; MGUS, monoclonal gammopathy of undetermined significance; MoAb, monoclonal antibody; MPN, myeloproliferative neoplasm; MRD, minimal residual disease; MZL, marginal zone lymphoma; NHL, non-Hodgkin lymphoma; NK, natural killer; NLPHL, nodular lymphocyte predominant Hodgkin lymphoma; PLL, prolymphocytic leukaemia; PNH, paroxysmal nocturnal haemoglobinuria; SLL, small lymphocytic lymphoma.

Immunophenotyping for Haematologists: Principles and Practice, First Edition. Barbara J. Bain and Mike Leach.
© 2021 John Wiley & Sons Ltd. Published 2021 by John Wiley & Sons Ltd.

Antibodies with CD numbers

CD1

A family of transmembrane proteins (CD1a, CD1b, CD1c, CD1d and CD1e) of which CD1a is used in immunophenotyping; expressed by cortical thymocytes; expressed by Langerhans cells, but not by interdigitating dendritic cells, follicular dendritic cells or macrophages; activated T cells may show cytoplasmic expression.

CD1a is expressed by blast cells of cortical T acute lymphoblastic leukaemia/lymphoblastic lymphoma (ALL/LL), in thymoma and in Langerhans cell histiocytosis; aberrantly expressed in some acute myeloid leukaemia (AML) and some B-cell neoplasms; less often expressed in chronic lymphocytic leukaemia (CLL) than by normal B cells, although in other B-cell neoplasms expression is often increased; expression in CLL is stronger among cases with unmutated *IGVH* genes; in bone marrow sections, CD1a stains the cytoplasm of Leishmania amastigotes.

Useful in the diagnosis of T-ALL and Langerhans cell histiocytosis; chimaeric antigen receptor T cells (CAR T cells) for use in T-ALL with CD1a expression are under development.

CD2

A pan-T marker, expressed by cortical and late thymocytes, mature T cells and most natural killer (NK) cells; expression by T cells increases with repeated antigenic stimulation; expressed by about 6% of normal peripheral blood B cells; not expressed by normal mast cells.

Expressed by blast cells of many cases of T-ALL/LL and cells of many leukaemias/lymphomas of mature T cells; expressed in around 10% of cases of AML, most often in acute promyelocytic leukaemia, particularly the microgranular variant, and AML with inv(16); expressed in about 16% of cases of CLL, about 55% of cases of follicular lymphoma, about 25% of cases of hairy cell leukaemia and about 30% of cases of diffuse large B-cell lymphoma (DLBCL); not usually expressed in mantle cell lymphoma; may be aberrantly expressed, together with CD25, by neoplastic mast cells and is particularly associated with systemic mastocytosis with an associated haematological neoplasm whereas the atypical mast cells associated with chronic eosinophilic leukaemia and a *FIP1L1-PDGFRA* fusion gene usually express CD25 but not CD2; sometimes expressed in blastic plasmacytoid dendritic cell neoplasm.

A monoclonal antibody (MoAb), siplizumab, has potential for therapy of T-cell lymphomas.

Useful in the diagnosis of T-lineage neoplasms and systemic mastocytosis; sometimes used for minimal residual disease (MRD) monitoring in AML.

CD3

A complex of at least five membrane-bound polypeptides (CD3γ, CD3δ, CD3ε, CD3ζ and CD3η) that are non-covalently associated with each other and with the T-cell receptor; the most specific T-cell marker; expressed on late thymocytes and mature T cells; CD3ε is expressed in the cytoplasm of NK cells and this can lead to positive reactions on immunohistochemistry.

CD3 is expressed by blast cells of many cases of T-ALL, with cytoplasmic expression only in cases with a more immature phenotype and surface membrane expression when the phenotype is more mature; expressed by neoplastic cells of many leukaemias/lymphomas of mature T cells but in some cases surface membrane expression is lost or is weak; the identification of cytoplasmic CD3 expression is the gold standard for defining T lineage; expression has been reported in a minority of cases of blastic plasmacytoid dendritic cell neoplasm.

Cytoplasmic and surface membrane CD3 expression is important in the diagnosis of T-ALL and for monitoring MRD; visilizumab is directed at the CD3 epsilon chain; blinatumomab is a bispecific anti-CD3 anti-CD19

MoAb that engages T cells and is of use in B-ALL, aggressive B-cell non-Hodgkin lymphoma (NHL) and B/myeloid mixed phenotype acute leukaemia; a bifunctional CD3-engaging, CD33-engaging, anti-PD-L1 (CD274)-delivering antibody has potential in AML; teplizumab can delay the development of type 1 diabetes mellitus in high-risk individuals.

CD4

Co-expressed with CD8 by common (cortical) thymocytes and expressed by a major subset of late thymocytes and mature T cells (helper/inducer) without co-expression of CD8; expressed by some NK cells (particularly in tissues and if activated); expressed by some immature myeloid cells including CD34-positive progenitor cells and subsets of eosinophils, basophils and neutrophils; expressed by promonocytes, monocytes, macrophages, Langerhans cells, follicular dendritic cells, plasmacytoid dendritic cells and myeloid dendritic cells; expressed by bone marrow endothelial cells; expressed by many mast cells.

Expressed by blast cells of many cases of T-ALL (usually together with CD8) and by cells of many leukaemias/lymphomas of mature T cells; sometimes expressed (more weakly) by blast cells in AML, particularly when there is monocytic differentiation, and in chronic myelomonocytic leukaemia (CMML); expressed in Langerhans cell histiocytosis; expressed, together with CD56, in blastic plasmacytoid dendritic cell neoplasm; expressed by mast cells in cutaneous mastocytosis and sometimes in systemic mastocytosis.

Useful in the diagnosis of T-lineage neoplasms and blastic plasmacytoid dendritic cell neoplasm, in MRD monitoring in T-ALL and AML and in monitoring T cell numbers in human immunodeficiency virus (HIV) infection; ibalizumab is a CD4 MoAb used in the treatment of multi-drug-resistant HIV infection; potentially a target of CAR T cells in T-NHL.

CD5

A pan-T marker, expressed by cortical and late thymocytes and some early thymocytes, by mature T cells, by a subset of normal B cells (found in the mantle zone of germinal centres and in small numbers in the blood); not expressed by NK cells; CD5-positive lymphocytes are expanded in various autoimmune diseases; downregulated on T lymphocytes in a minority of cases of infectious mononucleosis; may be downregulated on circulating T cells following bone marrow transplantation.

Expressed by blast cells of many cases of T-ALL, in many T-lineage leukaemias/lymphomas and in CLL and mantle cell lymphoma; expressed in a small minority of cases of DLBCL, correlating with an activated B-cell-like phenotype; can be aberrantly expressed in AML; expressed in about 12% of carcinomas and in a significant minority of mesotheliomas.

Important in the diagnosis of CLL and mantle cell lymphoma; sometimes used for MRD monitoring in AML.

CD7

A pan-T marker but not T-cell specific, expressed by pluripotent haemopoietic stem cells, some common lymphoid progenitor cells, thymocytes, NK cells and the majority of mature T cells; not expressed by a small subset of suppressor T cells; expressed by a subset of immature myeloid cells; downregulated on T cells in infectious mononucleosis, inflammatory dermatoses and rheumatoid arthritis.

Expressed by blast cells of T-ALL, leukaemic cells of T prolymphocytic leukaemia (PLL) and, much less often, the cells of other T-lineage leukaemias/lymphomas; it is expressed by blast cells of a significant minority (*c.* 15−20%) of cases of AML and, if cases with *CEBPA* mutation are excluded, is associated with a worse prognosis; may be expressed in blastic plasmacytoid dendritic cell neoplasm; expressed in about a fifth of carcinomas and in about half of mesotheliomas.

Useful in distinguishing T-PLL (expression retained) from other neoplasms of mature T cells (expression often lost) and for monitoring MRD in AML.

CD8

Expressed by cortical thymocytes together with CD4; expressed by a subset of late thymocytes and mature T cells without co-expression of CD4, these being cytotoxic/suppressor T cells that recognise antigen in the context of class I major histocompatibility complex antigens; expressed by macrophages but not osteoclasts; expressed by NK cells; mast cells and dendritic cells may be positive.

Expressed in most cases of large granular lymphocytic leukaemia and in a smaller proportion of cases of other T-lineage leukaemias/lymphomas, including some T-PLL (either alone or with CD4); expressed in about 2% of cases of B-cell leukaemia/lymphoma, particularly CLL/small lymphocytic lymphoma (SLL); expressed in some angiosarcomas.

Useful in the diagnosis of T-lineage neoplasms and T-ALL and for MRD monitoring in T-ALL.

CD9

Expressed by haemopoietic stem cells, megakaryocyte progenitors, megakaryocytes, platelets, early B cells, activated B and T cells, plasma cells, monocytes, eosinophils, basophils, mast cells, immature dendritic cells, bone marrow stromal cells, endothelial cells, neural and glial cells of the brain and peripheral nerves, vascular and cardiac smooth muscle and epithelial cells.

Expressed in B-ALL, in hypergranular promyelocytic leukaemia and acute basophilic leukaemia and less often in other types of AML and thus useful if acute basophilic leukaemia is suspected; expressed by neoplastic mast cells; may be weakly expressed by neuroblastoma cells; may be expressed in melanoma and breast cancer.

CD10

'Common ALL antigen', expressed by a subset of normal B-cell progenitors including B cells in germinal centres and 'haematogones' – non-neoplastic immature B-lineage lymphoid cells that are seen particularly in the bone marrow of children; expressed by a minority (less than 10%) of circulating B cells in neonates; expressed by a subset of mature T cells and B cells including germinal centre B cells and some follicular helper T cells; expressed by some plasma cells, neutrophils (but not eosinophils) and by monocytes and macrophages; also expressed by bone marrow stromal cells and by a number of non-haemopoietic/non-lymphoid cells; expression by neutrophils can be reduced in infection including HIV infection, following granulocyte colony-stimulating factor (G-CSF) administration, in adult onset chronic granulomatous disease and in myelodysplastic syndromes (MDS) and myelodysplastic/myeloproliferative neoplasms (MDS/MPN).

Expressed in the majority of cases of B-ALL, more weakly in about a third of cases of T-ALL, in many cases of follicular lymphoma (but often negative in the bone marrow unless there is follicle formation) and in a lower proportion of cases of other B-NHL including primary mediastinal large B-cell lymphoma (25–40% of cases) and blastoid mantle cell lymphoma; expressed in the germinal centre B-cell-like subset of DLBCL; usually expressed in Burkitt lymphoma and is expressed in 10–20% of cases of hairy cell leukaemia; expressed in angioimmunoblastic T-cell lymphoma and follicular T-cell lymphoma; expressed by a subset of myeloma cells in some patients and more often expressed in plasma cell leukaemia; expressed in a significant proportion of many non-haemopoietic tumours including renal carcinoma.

Useful in the diagnosis of B-ALL, follicular lymphoma, germinal centre B-cell-like DLBCL, Burkitt lymphoma, angioimmunoblastic T-cell lymphoma and follicular T-cell lymphoma; can be used for monitoring MRD in ALL since expression is homogeneous and bright whereas it is heterogeneous on haematogones.

CD11a

α chain that forms a heterodimer with CD18; expressed by all leucocytes; expressed by macrophages but not osteoclasts; expression is absent in leucocyte adhesion deficiency type I, a congenital disorder characterised by neutrophilia and recurrent bacterial infections due to deficiency of CD18.

Expressed (as the heterodimer with CD18) in some cases of multiple myeloma; may be expressed (with CD18) in follicular lymphoma but not expressed in CLL; may be expressed in AML, correlating with a worse prognosis; usually negative in acute promyelocytic leukaemia and in acute megakaryoblastic leukaemia and transient abnormal myelopoiesis of Down's syndrome.

CD11b

α chain that forms a heterodimer with CD18; a complement receptor expressed by promonocytes, mature monocytes and macrophages but not osteoclasts; expressed by NK cells; expressed from the myelocyte stage onwards in the neutrophil lineage; expressed more weakly by mature neutrophils than by monocytes but expression is increased when neutrophils are activated, for example, by the administration of G-CSF; on monocytes, CD11b is expressed more strongly than CD15 whereas the reverse is true of maturing neutrophils; sometimes expressed by basophils and variably expressed by mast cells; expressed by eosinophils; expressed by a subset of B cells (CD5-positive activated B cells) and a subset of T cells (cytotoxic CD8-positive T cells); expressed, together with high levels of CD11c, by a subset of mature thymic dendritic cells; expression is absent in leucocyte adhesion deficiency type I.

Expressed in many cases of AML, particularly those with monocytic differentiation; often expressed in AML with *NPM1* mutation;

usually negative in acute promyelocytic leukaemia, a CD34-negative, human leucocyte antigen (HLA)-DR-negative, CD11b-negative immunophenotype being useful in the diagnosis of this condition; occasionally expressed in CLL; expressed in hairy cell leukaemia; expressed in chronic lymphoproliferative disorder of NK cells.

Useful in the diagnosis of AML and T-cell large granular lymphocytic leukaemia and for monitoring MRD in AML.

CD11c

α chain that forms a heterodimer with CD18; expressed by promonocytes, monocytes, macrophages, NK cells and neutrophils (more weakly than by monocytes); not expressed by osteoclasts; expressed by mast cells but weakly if at all by basophils; expressed by myeloid but not lymphoid dendritic cells; expressed, together with CD11b, by a subset of mature thymic dendritic cells; expressed by some T cells and B cells including activated T and B cells; expression is absent in leucocyte adhesion deficiency type I.

May be expressed in AML, including AML with t(8;21) and when there is monocytic differentiation; usually negative in acute promyelocytic leukaemia; strongly expressed by hairy cells and expressed in some cases of hairy cell leukaemia variant, B-PLL and splenic marginal zone lymphoma (MZL); expressed in about 40% of cases of CLL when expression is weaker than in hairy cell leukaemia and is prognostically adverse; not usually expressed in other lymphoproliferative disorders; more often and more strongly expressed by the neoplastic cells of systemic mastocytosis than by normal mast cells.

Useful in the diagnosis of AML and hairy cell leukaemia.

CD13

Strongly expressed by CD34-positive stem cells and CD117-positive granulocyte precursors (promyelocytes) and is then downregulated on myelocytes and upregulated again on neutrophils; expressed by eosinophils (more strongly than by neutrophils) and basophils; expressed by early committed monocyte progenitors; expressed by dendritic cells, macrophages and osteoclasts; expressed by mast cells and their precursors; expressed by some plasma cells; expressed by endothelial cells when there is angiogenesis but not expressed by other endothelial cells; expressed by bone marrow stromal cells and in a number of non-haemopoietic tissues.

Expressed by blast cells in the majority of cases of AML; expressed by some myeloma cells; aberrantly expressed in about half of cases of anaplastic large cell lymphoma (ALCL); may be aberrantly expressed in ALL, more often in B-ALL (particularly Ph (*BCR-ABL1*)-positive, *KMT2A* rearranged and *ETV6-RUNX1*-positive ALL) than T-ALL, and expressed less often in mature B-lineage lymphoid neoplasms; may be expressed by neoplastic plasma cells; expressed in some non-haemopoietic neoplasms.

Useful in the diagnosis of AML and for MRD monitoring; useful for MRD monitoring in B-ALL, in which aberrant expression suggests the above genetic subtypes; CAR T cells applicable to treatment of AML are under development.

CD14

A glycosylphosphatidylinositol (GPI)-anchored cell surface glycoprotein; expressed by monocytes and weakly by macrophages and neutrophils; not expressed by osteoclasts, basophils or mast cells; expressed by circulating myeloid dendritic cells and some immature tissue dendritic cells.

Expressed in many cases of AML, particularly those showing monocytic differentiation but typically absent in acute monoblastic leukaemia; variably expressed by promonocytes; expressed by monocytes in CMML; can be aberrantly expressed by maturing cells of neutrophil lineage in MDS and MDS/MPN; aberrant expression of CD14 in CLL has been associated

with a worse prognosis; expressed in the majority of cases of Langerhans cell histiocytosis.

Useful in the diagnosis of AML and Langerhans cell histiocytosis; sometimes used for MRD monitoring in AML; as CD14 is GPI anchored, expression is lost by monocytes in patients with paroxysmal nocturnal haemoglobinuria (PNH).

CD15

Expressed by maturing cells of monocyte lineage (60% of monocytes) and more weakly by maturing cells of neutrophil (90%) and eosinophil lineages, from the promyelocyte stage onwards; expression by eosinophils is weaker than neutrophil expression; not expressed by basophils or mast cells; CD15s is the sialylated form, which is the ligand of E and P selectins (CD62E and CD62P); MoAbs detect either the sialylated form, CD15s, or the non-sialylated form, CD15; Rambam–Hasharon syndrome is an autosomal recessive inborn error of fucose metabolism associated with a lack of sialylation of CD15, with an immune defect designated leucocyte adhesion deficiency type II in which the CD15s-negative neutrophils fail to migrate normally into tissues leading to neutrophilia and recurrent infections.

Expressed by the blast cells of many cases of AML, particularly if there is monocytic differentiation or *KMT2A* rearrangement; weakly expressed in acute promyelocytic leukaemia, in contrast to strong expression by normal promyelocytes; can be aberrantly expressed in pro-B-ALL, particularly with *KMT2A* rearrangement; expressed by Reed–Sternberg cells and mononuclear Hodgkin cells in classical Hodgkin lymphoma (but not expressed in nodular lymphocyte predominant Hodgkin lymphoma (NLPHL)); expressed by cells of a small proportion of NHL including some mycosis fungoides and other T-cell lymphomas but not ALCL, which is usually CD15−; often expressed by carcinoma cells.

Useful in the diagnosis of AML and, together with CD30, in the histological diagnosis of classical Hodgkin lymphoma; useful for MRD monitoring in B-ALL and AML.

CD16

A GPI-anchored integral membrane protein of neutrophils, part of the low-affinity Fcγ receptor, FcRIII, which mediates phagocytosis and antibody-dependent cell-mediated cytotoxicity; includes CD16a and CD16b, which differ somewhat in structure and are expressed by a somewhat different range of cells; expressed by mature NK cells (CD16a), when it is not GPI-linked (but not NK precursors or immature NK cells), some T cells (CD16a), neutrophils (from metamyelocyte stage onwards) (CD16b and more weakly CD16a), activated monocytes and macrophages (CD16a) but not osteoclasts; not expressed or expressed weakly by eosinophils unless they are activated; not expressed by basophils or mast cells; constitutive expression by neutrophils is cytoplasmic with transient surface membrane expression occurring when they are exposed to complement; expression by neutrophils is reduced by administration of G-CSF.

CD16 is expressed in a significant minority of cases of AML; CD16a is a fairly specific but not very sensitive marker of monocytic differentiation; expressed in some NK-cell neoplasms, specifically aggressive NK cell leukaemia/lymphoma and some cases of nasal-type NK-cell leukaemia/lymphoma; not expressed in blastic plasmacytoid dendritic cell neoplasm.

Useful for characterising monocyte subsets and for the diagnosis of large granular lymphocytic leukaemia and NK neoplasms; lack of expression by neutrophils can be used in the diagnosis of PNH and in this circumstance testing should not be delayed as expression is lost on ageing of cells.

CD19

Expressed by B lymphocytes and their precursors, one of the earliest of the B-lineage-associated antigens to be expressed; expressed weakly by most normal plasma cells; expressed by follicular dendritic cells; cytoplasmic expression, together with expression of CD79a, is indicative of B-cell lineage.

Expressed in the majority of cases of B-ALL and B-lineage leukaemias and lymphomas including NLPHL, but not in primary effusion lymphoma or ALK-positive large B-cell lymphoma; reduced expression is common in DLBCL; not usually expressed in myeloma; sometimes aberrantly expressed in AML, particularly in cases with t(8;21) or t(9;22), and MDS; expressed at low levels in some T-ALL.

Can be the target of CAR T cells (e.g. tisagenlecleucel and axicabtagene ciloleucel) in B-ALL, CLL and B-NHL including follicular lymphoma and DLBCL (but in one study in DLBCL effectiveness was not related to expression, or the strength of expression, of the antigen); CAR T cells are also potentially applicable to autoimmune diseases; CD19 can be the target of CAR NK cells in NHL and CLL; blinatumomab is a bispecific anti-CD3 anti-CD19 MoAb that engages T cells and is of use in B-ALL; an antibody–drug conjugate, loncastuximab, has potential in the treatment of DLBCL.

Useful in the diagnosis of B-lineage neoplasms; aberrant expression (sometimes with CD56) in AML suggests possible t(8;21); useful for MRD monitoring in AML.

CD20

Expressed by B lymphocytes and their precursors but not by the earliest identifiable precursors; upregulated with B-cell activation; not expressed by most normal plasma cells; weakly expressed by a T-cell subset; can be expressed by follicular dendritic cells.

Expressed in some cases (about 40%) of B-ALL but not in pro-B-ALL; expressed in the majority of cases of B-lineage leukaemias and lymphomas but more weakly expressed in CLL than in other mature B-cell neoplasms; expressed in NLPHL; strongly expressed in hairy cell leukaemia; not expressed in primary effusion lymphoma or ALK-positive large B-cell lymphoma; expression may be reduced in DLBCL; expressed in a minority of cases of multiple myeloma but more often expressed in plasma cell leukaemia; CD20 expression in multiple myeloma shows some correlation with small, mature myeloma cells and with the presence of t(11;14) and cyclin D1 expression; expressed in NLPHL and expressed, more weakly, by the neoplastic cells of 30–40% of classical Hodgkin lymphoma; occasionally expressed in AML and rarely in T-NHL; downregulated on B cells after rituximab treatment.

Monoclonal antibodies (rituximab, veltuzumab, ocaratuzumab, ocrelizumab, ofatumumab, ublituximab and obinutuzumab) are widely used for therapy of B-cell neoplasms and are similarly applicable to NLPHL; in B-ALL, CD20 is upregulated by corticosteroid therapy, which may increase the effectiveness of MoAb therapy; rituximab can replace chemotherapy in early stage NLPHL; the radiopharmaceuticals, ^{90}Y-ibritumomab tiuxetan, ^{90}Y-rituximab and ^{131}I-tositumomab, are similarly applicable to B-cell NHL and NLPHL; mosunetuzumab is a bispecific CD3 CD20 MoAb applicable to B-lineage lymphomas; rituximab is also of value as an immunosuppressive agent, for example, in thrombotic thrombocytopenic purpura, chronic cold haemagglutinin disease and refractory autoimmune thrombocytopenic purpura; CD20 can be the target of CAR T cells.

Useful in the diagnosis of B-lineage neoplasms.

See also FMC7.

CD21

A complement receptor, expressed by a subset of normal B cells including mantle zone and marginal zone lymphocytes but not follicular centre cells; not expressed by B-cell precursors; downregulated with B-cell activation; expressed weakly by a T-cell subset; expressed by follicular dendritic cells including those in the bone marrow, helping to distinguish them from interdigitating dendritic cells, Langerhans cells and macrophages.

Expressed in most cases of CLL and in about 50% of cases of B-NHL but expression by CLL cells is weaker than that of normal B cells; weakly expressed by hairy cells; expressed in some cases of T-ALL; expressed by neoplastic cells in a minority of cases of Hodgkin lymphoma; expressed in some cases of follicular dendritic cell sarcoma (but not in histiocytic sarcoma, Langerhans cell histiocytosis or interdigitating cell tumour).

Useful in immunohistochemistry for demonstrating the follicular dendritic cell network in germinal centres.

CD22

Siglec-2, sialic acid-binding immunoglobulin-like lectin 2, expressed on the surface membrane of B lymphocytes and in the cytoplasm of their precursors; downregulated on B-cell activation; variably expressed by mast cells; expression by basophils and monocytes is detected with some but not all MoAb; not expressed by plasma cells; expressed by normal and neoplastic plasmacytoid dendritic cells but in the latter the rate of detection varies between different anti-CD22 clones.

Expressed in the cytoplasm of the blast cells of most cases of B-ALL but less frequently on the surface membrane; expressed on the surface membrane of cells of most cases of B-NHL and hairy cell leukaemia (strong expression) but not on the cells of CLL in which expression is weak or absent; expressed in NLPHL.

A MoAb linked to a toxin (moxetumomab pasudotox) is efficacious in hairy cell leukaemia, in NHL and in some cases of ALL; pinatuzumab vedotin is of potential value in DLBCL and follicular lymphoma; when expressed in B-ALL and non-Hodgkin lymphoma, CD22 can be the target of CAR T cells; inotuzumab ozogamicin, a MoAb linked to a toxin, has a role in relapsed/refractory B-ALL and in AML; ^{90}Y-epratuzumab tetraxetan is a radiopharmaceutical.

Useful in the diagnosis of B-lineage neoplasms; sometimes used for MRD monitoring in AML and CLL.

CD23

A low-affinity Fcε receptor (FcεRII); expressed weakly by B cells in the follicular mantle and strongly by activated germinal centre B cells; expressed weakly by 30–40% of peripheral blood B cells, more strongly by activated B cells; expressed by a subset of CD4-positive T cells, neutrophils, eosinophils, monocytes, macrophages (particularly when activated), Langerhans cells, follicular dendritic cells including those in the bone marrow, platelets and some bone marrow stromal cells; has been reported to be expressed less often by the cells of polyclonal B-cell lymphocytosis than by normal B cells; expressed by epithelial cells, for example, of stomach, intestine and lung; CD23-positive cells are rare on immunohistochemical staining of normal bone marrow.

Expressed in most cases of CLL/SLL, most strongly in proliferation centres, but in only a minority of cases of B-PLL and other categories of B-NHL; expressed more often in low grade lymphoma than in high grade and more often in follicular lymphoma, lymphoplasmacytic lymphoma and mantle cell lymphoma than most other B-NHL; expressed in about a quarter of cases of mantle cell lymphoma; usually expressed in mediastinal large B-cell lymphoma; expressed in about 10% of cases of multiple myeloma, expression correlating with abnormalities of chromosome 11, particularly t(11;14)(q13;q32), and with plasma cell leukaemia; staining of follicular dendritic cells is useful for the demonstration of a follicular pattern in lymphomas; can be aberrantly expressed in AML; can be expressed by eosinophils in chronic eosinophilic leukaemia associated with *PDGFRA* rearrangement.

Useful in the diagnosis of B-lineage neoplasms, particularly for the recognition of CLL; useful in immunohistochemistry for demonstrating the follicular dendritic cell network in germinal centres.

CD24

A GPI-anchored cell surface glycoprotein, expressed by B lymphocytes and their precursors, by activated T lymphocytes, by neutrophils, by eosinophils and by some follicular dendritic cells; expressed by some epithelial cells.

CD24 is expressed by the blast cells of the majority of cases of B-ALL but not those associated with a cytogenetic rearrangement with an 11q23 breakpoint; expressed in the majority of cases of B-lineage leukaemia/lymphoma and by blast cells of some cases of AML, particularly when there is monocytic differentiation for which it is a fairly specific but not very sensitive marker; weakly expressed on hairy cells; expressed by carcinoma cells including cells of small cell carcinoma of the lung; CD24 is lacking from the neutrophils in PNH.

The main role for assessing CD24 expression is in the diagnosis of PNH.

CD25

The α chain of interleukin (IL) 2 receptor (IL2R); high affinity IL2R is a complex of CD25 with CD122 and CD132; expressed by activated B and T cells (particularly the Th2 subset) including HIV-infected T cells; expressed by the majority of CD4-positive regulatory T cells and by some regulatory CD4-positive and CD8-positive thymocytes; expressed by monocytes and macrophages (particularly when activated) and by the cells of polyclonal B-cell lymphocytosis; sometimes expressed by basophils but not by normal mast cells; T lymphocytes that coexpress CD4 and CD25 inhibit immune responses to both foreign and self antigens; on immunohistochemical staining, there is positivity in megakaryocytes and adipocytes.

CD25 is expressed in hairy cell leukaemia, in the great majority of cases of adult T-cell leukaemia/lymphoma (ATLL) and sometimes in other high-grade lymphomas including ALCL and DLBCL; can also be expressed by a large proportion of T cells of individuals carrying the human T-cell lymphotropic virus 1 (HTLV-1) who do not have ATLL; expressed in some patients with CLL, expression being linked to a worse prognosis; expressed in lymphoplasma-cytic lymphoma and in many cases of B-PLL; expressed by mononuclear Hodgkin cells and Reed–Sternberg cells in classical Hodgkin lymphoma; may be expressed by eosinophils in chronic eosinophilic leukaemia associated with *FIP1L1-PDGFRA*; expressed by neoplastic mast cells, both in systemic mastocytosis and in acute mast cell leukaemia and also by atypi-cal mast cells of chronic eosinophilic leukae-mia associated with a *FIP1L1-PDGFRA* fusion gene; expression is reported in a quarter to two-thirds of cases of AML and is associated with a worse prognosis; expressed in some cases of B-ALL and in a small minority of T-ALL cases.

Useful in the diagnosis of hairy cell leukae-mia, ATLL and systemic mastocytosis; elevated soluble CD25 is one of the criteria used in the diagnosis of haemophagocytic lymphohistio-cytosis (HLH); MoAbs, daclizumab and basiliximab have not been found to be thera-peutically very useful; daclizumab has now been withdrawn from the market, but basi-liximab conjugated to Y[101] is now under eval-uation; camidanlumab tesirine, a MoAb conjugated to a toxin, also has potential for therapy in classical Hodgkin lymphoma and other CD30-positive neoplasms.

CD26

A costimulatory molecule for T-cell activa-tion that is upregulated on T-cell activation; expressed by mature thymocytes, activated T cells (particularly CD4-positive T cells), B cells, NK cells, macrophages, renal proximal tubule cells, fibroblasts, some epithelial cells includ-ing small intestinal epithelial cells, prostatic cells, biliary canalicular cells, brain, heart, skeletal muscle, endothelial cells and splenic sinus lining cells; expressed by more than 50% of peripheral blood lymphocytes in healthy people including expression by more than 70% of CD4-positive T cells.

Expressed by leukaemic stem cells in chronic myeloid leukaemia (CML) but not by normal stem cells or leukaemic stem cells in other hae-matological neoplasms; lymphoma cells in mycosis fungoides/Sézary syndrome and other types of T-cell lymphoma may fail to express CD26; in other T-cell lymphomas, for example, T-PLL and ALCL, expression is retained and is homogeneous, in contrast to the heterogene-ous expression of normal T cells; usually strongly expressed in hairy cell leukaemia, sometimes expressed in CLL and multiple myeloma and negative in follicular lymphoma and mantle cell lymphoma.

Lack of expression of CD26 has been found useful in the identification of circulating neo-plastic cells in mycosis fungoides and Sézary syndrome but there can also be a lack of expression in reactive conditions; uniform expression of CD26 can be a sign of T-cell clonality.

CD27

A costimulatory molecule for B and T cells; expressed by medullary thymocytes, some T cells, NK cells and somatically mutated memory B cells (but not immature or mature but naïve B cells); an early activation marker on T cells; expressed by normal plasma cells.

Often expressed by neoplastic B cells with the phenotype of a mature B cell, including most cases of CLL, three quarters of cases of follicular lymphoma, two thirds of cases of DLBCL and most cases of splenic MZL; expres-sion is similar whether the leukaemia/lym-phoma is apparently derived from naïve or memory B cells; not expressed on B-lineage lymphoblasts; not expressed in hairy cell leu-kaemia; expression by myeloma cells is weaker than by normal plasma cells; not expressed in about a third of cases of myeloma and half of relapsed cases; more likely to be expressed by plasma cells in monoclonal gammopathy of undetermined significance (MGUS) than by myeloma cells; expressed by the cells of poly-clonal B-cell lymphocytosis, which may repre-sent an expansion of memory B cells.

CD28

A costimulatory marker on T cells; expressed by mature thymocytes, most T cells and activated B cells; expressed by long-lived bone marrow plasma cells.

Expressed in about a third of cases of multiple myeloma and may be strongly expressed; less often expressed in MGUS; expression in myeloma is prognostically adverse.

CD30

Expressed by activated B cells and T cells, NK cells, eosinophils and monocytes; expressed on Th2, but not Th1, T cells; on T cells is a late activation marker; weakly expressed by late erythroid cells and late cells of neutrophil lineage; expressed by plasma cells; not expressed by normal mast cells.

Strongly expressed by cells carrying HIV, HTLV-1 or Epstein–Barr virus (EBV); expressed in human herpesvirus 8 (HHV8)-associated Castleman disease; can be expressed by large T cells in reactive conditions, for example, herpes simplex infection, leading to simulation of lymphoma; strongly expressed by Hodgkin cells and Reed–Sternberg cells in classical Hodgkin lymphoma; strongly expressed by the lymphoma cells of ALCL including primary cutaneous ALCL, anaplastic variant of DLBCL, primary effusion lymphoma, primary mediastinal B-cell lymphoma and plasmablastic lymphoma, and can be weakly expressed in other types of large cell NHL; in one study was expressed in 14% of cases of DLBCL, both germinal centre B-cell-like and activated B-cell-like categories, and correlated with a better prognosis (perhaps particularly in germinal centre B-cell-like DLBCL); in non-germinal-centre type DLBCL, is more likely to be positive in EBV-positive cases; expressed in EBV-positive follicular lymphoma; expressed in about a third of cases of transformed mycosis fungoides; sometimes expressed in enteropathy-associated T-cell lymphoma; expressed in lymphomatoid papulosis; expressed in cutaneous intralymphatic CD30-positive T-cell lymphoma; can be expressed in aggressive systemic mastocytosis and mast cell leukaemia; expressed in some non-haemopoietic tumours.

There is therapeutic value for CD30-directed MoAbs in classical Hodgkin lymphoma, ALCL, primary effusion lymphoma, CD30-positive mycosis fungoides, ATLL and other CD30-positive lymphomas, and also some CD30-negative lymphomas; therapeutic antibodies include humanised monoclonal anti-CD30, CD30 antibodies conjugated to a cytotoxic drug such as auristatin (brentuximab vedotin) or to a radioisotope such as ^{131}I, and natural killer cell-activating bi-specific CD16-CD30 and CD64-CD30 antibodies; potentially a target of CAR T cells in classical (but not nodular lymphocyte-predominant) Hodgkin lymphoma; CD30 MoAbs linked to magnetic microbeads have been used experimentally for the isolation of mononuclear Hodgkin cells and Reed–Sternberg cells.

Important, together with CD15, in the histological diagnosis of classical Hodgkin lymphoma, in the differential diagnosis of large B-cell lymphomas and in the diagnosis of anaplastic large T-cell lymphoma.

CD31

A cell surface glycoprotein, platelet/endothelial cell adhesion molecule 1 (PECAM-1), expressed strongly by endothelial cells, including lymphatic endothelial cells and including those of the bone marrow; expressed more weakly by platelets, megakaryocytes and megakaryoblasts, haemopoietic progenitors, monocytes, macrophages, osteoclasts, neutrophils, eosinophils, Langerhans cells, NK cells, a subset of T cells, a subset of B cells (particularly marginal zone B cells) and plasma cells.

Expressed by plasma cells in MGUS and in plasmacytic myeloma but much less often in plasmablastic myeloma and plasma cell leukaemia; may be expressed in CLL; expressed in some cases of ALL and AML; expressed in blastic plasmacytoid dendritic cell neoplasm; expressed in benign and malignant tumours of endothelial origin.

Used in immunohistochemistry for identifying tumours of endothelial origin.

CD32

A low-affinity immunoglobulin (Ig)G receptor – FcγRII; expressed by monocytes, macrophages, Langerhans cells, neutrophils, eosinophils, platelets, mast cells and B cells; expressed by NK cells of some individuals; neutrophil expression is increased by the administration of G-CSF; there are two different receptors detected by antibodies of this cluster, FcγRIIa (CD32A, expressed by neutrophils, eosinophils, macrophages and platelets) and FcγRIIb (CD32B, expressed by neutrophils, macrophages, mast cells and B cells).

Often expressed in AML, more often when there is monocytic differentiation but not with sufficient specificity for this to be diagnostically useful; CD32b is highly expressed by clonal plasma cells in light chain-associated amyloidosis, providing a potential target for MoAb therapy.

CD33

Siglec-3, sialic acid-binding immunoglobulin-like lectin 3; expressed by myeloblasts, promyelocytes and myelocytes and expressed weakly by mature neutrophils; reduced expression can result from a polymorphism; expressed more strongly by monocytes than by neutrophils, expression by monocytes increasing with maturation; expressed by macrophages; expressed by some dendritic cells, which are viewed as being of myeloid origin, but not by others viewed as being of lymphoid origin; sometimes expressed by basophils and usually expressed by mast cells; expression by eosinophils is weak; expressed by some NK cells and some plasma cells.

Expressed by the blast cells of the majority of cases of AML; may be expressed in blastic plasmacytoid dendritic cell neoplasm; may be weakly expressed in ALL, more often in B-ALL than in T-ALL; expression is characteristic of the early precursor T-cell phenotype and in adults has been linked to an adverse prognosis; less often aberrantly expressed in mature lymphoid neoplasms; expressed by neoplastic mast cells; expressed in a minority of cases of myeloma.

Gemtuzumab ozogamicin (an anti-CD33 antibody linked to a DNA-intercalating cytotoxic agent), vadastuximab talirine (an anti-CD33 drug conjugate) and the anti-CD33 MoAb, lintuzumab, have been investigated for the treatment of AML but trials of vadastuximab talirine have been discontinued; CD33 MoAbs are potentially of use in early T-cell precursor ALL since two thirds of cases express the antigen; a bispecific CD3–CD33 MoAb is potentially of value in AML; a bifunctional CD3-engaging, CD33-engaging, anti-PD-L1 (CD274)-delivering antibody has potential in AML; CAR T cells for use in AML are under development.

Useful in the diagnosis and in MRD monitoring in AML; useful for MRD monitoring in B-ALL, in which aberrant expression suggests *BCR-ABL1* or *ETV6-RUNX1*.

CD34

A cell adhesion molecule expressed by lymphoid and haemopoietic stem cells; expressed by no more than 1–2% of normal bone marrow cells; expressed by myeloblasts but not promyelocytes; expressed by type I haematogones (normal B-cell precursors); expressed by some proerythroblasts and by early megaloblasts; expressed by the earliest identifiable mast cell precursors; may be expressed by megakaryocytes in MDS and in megaloblastic anaemia; expressed by non-lymphatic endothelial cells including those of the bone marrow.

Expressed by the blast cells of most cases of AML (but monoblasts are generally negative); a CD34-negative, HLA-DR-negative, CD11b-negative immunophenotype is useful in the diagnosis of acute promyelocytic leukaemia; more often expressed in the variant form of acute promyelocytic leukaemia than in the classical hypergranular form; usually negative in *NPM1*-mutated AML; expressed by blast cells in MDS; may be expressed by megakaryocytes in myeloid neoplasms; expressed in about 70% of cases of B-ALL (pro-B and common but not pre-B) and some cases of T-ALL; expressed in Kaposi's sarcoma, gastrointestinal stromal tumour and dermatofibrosarcoma protuberans.

Useful for the identification, enumeration and sorting of haemopoietic stem cells and blast cells; leukaemic stem cells are identified as CD34+CD38−; important in diagnosis and MRD monitoring in AML, B-ALL and T-ALL; lack of expression in AML is useful for suggesting a diagnosis of acute promyelocytic leukaemia or *NPM1*-mutated AML; useful in the diagnosis of MDS, with immunohistochemistry aiding in the identification of abnormal localisation of immature precursors (ALIP); possibly useful in the diagnosis of congenital macrothrombocytopenia due to *GFI1B* mutation, in which CD34 is expressed on platelets; useful for identification of the endothelium of capillaries and sinusoids in bone marrow sections and for the diagnosis of Kaposi's sarcoma.

CD35

A complement receptor, expressed by erythroid cells (weakly), neutrophils, eosinophils, basophils, monocytes, macrophages, B cells and 10–15% of T cells; expressed by some normal mast cells; expressed by follicular dendritic cells but not Langerhans cells or interdigitating dendritic cells.

Often expressed in AML, particularly when there is monocytic differentiation; more often expressed by neoplastic mast cells both in systemic mastocytosis and in acute mast cell leukaemia than by normal mast cells and more strongly expressed; expressed in NHL but not usually expressed in CLL; expressed in follicular dendritic cell tumours (but not in histiocytic sarcoma, Langerhans cell histiocytosis or interdigitating cell tumours).

Useful in immunohistochemistry for demonstrating the follicular dendritic cell network in germinal centres.

CD36

Platelet glycoprotein IV, thrombospondin receptor; expressed by megakaryoblasts, megakaryocytes and platelets; expressed by most erythroblasts; expressed by reticulocytes, fetal red cells, monocytes, macrophages, some plasmacytoid dendritic cells, microvascular endothelium and some other non-haemopoietic cells; expression by monocytes is stronger than by monocyte precursors; CD36 deficiency is present in at least 2–3% of Japanese, Thais and Africans but in less than 0.3% of Caucasians and can be involved in some cases of refractoriness to transfusion of HLA-matched platelets and some cases of alloimmune neonatal thrombocytopenia.

CD36 is expressed by megakaryoblasts in acute megakaryoblastic leukaemia; expressed in pure erythroid leukaemia; expressed by cells of monocyte lineage; upregulated in precursor cells in CML.

Useful in the diagnosis of acute megakaryoblastic leukaemia; sometimes used for MRD monitoring in AML.

CD37

A member of the transmembrane 4 or tetraspanin superfamily of proteins, involved in signal transduction; strongly expressed by mature B cells but expressed only weakly by plasma cells, T cells, neutrophils, monocytes, macrophages and dendritic cells; may be expressed by pre-B lymphoblasts.

Strongly expressed in CLL and B-NHL; not expressed in multiple myeloma or classical Hodgkin lymphoma; sometimes expressed in T-cell lymphomas including some angioimmunoblastic T-cell lymphomas, some ALK-negative anaplastic large cell lymphomas, some cutaneous T-cell lymphomas and some peripheral T-cell lymphomas, not otherwise specified.

Strong expression was previously used as a B-cell marker but more specific markers are now preferred; however, anti-CD37 CAR T cells are potentially effective in CD37-expressing B- and T-cell lymphomas and testing is therefore indicated if this therapy is being considered; this is particularly so for T-cell lymphomas when only a proportion of cases are positive; in T-cell lymphomas there is an advantage that normal T cells are spared; can be used for monitoring MRD in the uncommon cases of ALL that are positive since haematogones are negative; otlertuzumab, a fully humanised, monospecific anti-CD37 MoAb shows moderate activity in CLL; a radio-labelled MoAb is under trial in follicular lymphoma; MoAb therapy also has potential in DLBCL without *CD37* mutation.

CD38

Expressed by thymic cells, haemopoietic stem cells (being expressed later than CD34), B-cell precursors, germinal centre B cells, some activated circulating B cells, plasma cells (strongly), early T cells, some mature T cells (most tissue T cells but a minority of peripheral blood T cells); expressed by naïve CD45RA+ T cells but not CD45RO+ memory T cells; expressed by activated T cells, activated NK cells, a subset of monocytes (but not tissue macrophages), osteoclasts, basophils (more strongly than by neutrophils and eosinophils) but not mast cells, red cells, erythroid precursors or platelets; expressed by many non-haemopoietic cells.

Expressed by myeloma cells but more weakly than by normal plasma cells (expression correlating with a worse prognosis), in primary effusion lymphoma, in some cases of splenic MZL, in plasmablastic lymphoma, in lymphoplasmacytic lymphoma, in some cases of CLL (correlating with clonal origin from a less mature cell – unmutated *IGVH* genes – and with worse prognosis); expressed in a minority of cases of mantle cell lymphoma; in follicular lymphoma is expressed more weakly than by germinal centre cells in follicular hyperplasia; often expressed in AML and ALL; often expressed in neoplasms of mature T and NK cells; usually expressed in the acute form of ATLL; leukaemic stem cells are CD34+ but CD38−.

A MoAb, daratumumab, has therapeutic potential in myeloma and light-chain-associated amyloidosis and possibly also primary effusion lymphoma, AML, T-ALL and blastic plasmacytoid dendritic cell neoplasm; it has been used with success in refractory pure red cell aplasia following an ABO-incompatible haemopoietic stem cell transplant; isatuximab also has a role in myeloma treatment.

Useful for MRD monitoring in B-ALL, AML and myeloma and for prognostication in CLL.

CD40

Expressed by B cells and precursors, but not by the most immature B lymphoblasts; expressed weakly by plasma cells; expressed by CD34-positive haemopoietic progenitors, macrophages, platelets, endothelial cells, fibroblasts and some epithelial cells; variably expressed by normal and neoplastic mast cells; expressed weakly by immature dendritic cells, such as those in skin and other peripheral tissues, but expressed strongly by mature follicular dendritic cells in lymph nodes.

Expressed in B-ALL, CLL, some NHL, hairy cell leukaemia, multiple myeloma, the majority of cases of Langerhans cell histiocytosis and by Hodgkin/Reed–Sternberg cells in classical and lymphocyte predominant Hodgkin lymphoma; may be expressed in AML, expression correlating with a worse prognosis; expressed by carcinoma cells.

One monoclonal antibody, dacetuzumab, has therapeutic potential in CLL, myeloma and Hodgkin lymphoma but development of lucatumumab has been discontinued.

CD41a

Platelet glycoprotein IIb/IIIa complex (αIIbβ3 integrin); expressed by megakaryocytes and platelets; receptor for von Willebrand factor, fibronectin, fibrinogen and thrombospondin; not expressed by normal mast cells.

Expressed in acute megakaryoblastic leukaemia; may be expressed by neoplastic mast cells.

Useful in the diagnosis of acute megakaryoblastic leukaemia and Glanzmann's thrombasthenia (expression is reduced in most patients, but a non-functional protein is expressed in some patients).

CD41b

Platelet glycoprotein IIb; forms a heterodimer with β_3 integrin (CD61) with the heterodimer (αIIbβ3) being expressed by multipotent myeloid stem cells (CFU-GM), bipotent erythroid-megakaryocyte stem cells, megakaryocyte colony-forming cells (CFU-MK), megakaryocytes and platelets; mediates platelet adhesion to subendothelial matrix and platelet aggregation induced by fibrinogen, von Willebrand factor, thrombin, collagen, adenosine diphosphate (ADP) and adrenaline.

Expressed in acute megakaryoblastic leukaemia; may detect earlier cells than CD42b and CD61.

Useful in the diagnosis of acute megakaryoblastic leukaemia and Glanzmann's thrombasthenia.

CD42a

Platelet glycoprotein IX, expressed by megakaryocytes and platelets; the CD42a-d (or GpIb-IX-V) complex is the platelet receptor for von Willebrand factor and thrombin.

Expressed in acute megakaryoblastic leukaemia but is less sensitive than CD41 or CD61 as it is expressed later.

Useful in the diagnosis of acute megakaryoblastic leukaemia and Bernard–Soulier syndrome.

CD42b

Platelet glycoprotein Ibα, expressed by megakaryocytes and platelets; CD42a-d complex is the platelet receptor for von Willebrand factor and thrombin, the actual binding site being on the CD42b molecule; CD42b forms a heterodimer with CD42c with the heterodimer also being associated with CD42a and CD42d; not expressed by normal mast cells; expressed later than CD41 and CD61.

CD42b may be expressed, but usually only weakly, by megakaryoblasts of acute megakaryoblastic leukaemia; positivity in AML is usually the result of adherent platelets; megakaryocyte expression may be downregulated in MDS; may be expressed by neoplastic mast cells.

Useful in the diagnosis of acute megakaryoblastic leukaemia and for the immunohistochemical identification of megakaryocytes in MDS, myeloproliferative neoplasms (MPN), MDS/MPN and acute panmyelosis with myelofibrosis; useful in the diagnosis of Bernard–Soulier syndrome.

CD42c

Platelet glycoprotein Ibβ, expressed by megakaryocytes and platelets.

Useful in the diagnosis of Bernard–Soulier syndrome.

CD42d

Platelet glycoprotein V, expressed by megakaryocytes and platelets.

CD43

Expressed by T cells, a subset of B cells and occasionally by activated B cells; expressed by some B-cell precursors; expressed by myeloid cells including haemopoietic progenitors; expressed by neutrophils, monocytes, basophils and mast cells; expressed by plasmacytoid dendritic cells.

Expressed in T-ALL and T- and NK-cell lymphomas, in some cases of B-ALL and CLL/SLL, some B-PLL, mantle cell lymphoma and Burkitt lymphoma but rarely in follicular lymphoma, mainly in cases in large cell transformation; expressed in a small proportion of lymphoplasmacytic lymphomas and MZLs – mucosa-associated lymphoid tissues (MALT)-type lymphomas and splenic MZLs; expressed in blastic plasmacytoid dendritic cell neoplasm; often expressed in AML; expressed in Langerhans cell and histiocytic neoplasms; may be expressed by neoplastic mast cells; CD43 may be reduced on T cells in Wiskott–Aldrich syndrome.

CD44

Expressed by all blood cells except platelets; expressed by haemopoietic stem cells, plasma cells, macrophages, osteoclasts and mast cells; expressed by many non-haemopoietic cells.

Expressed in B-ALL, in CLL, in many NHLs, in multiple myeloma and in AML; expressed by neoplastic mast cells.

CAR T cells for use in AML are under development.

CD45

The common leucocyte antigen, expressed by all haemopoietic cells except mature red cells and their immediate precursors; expressed by megakaryocytes and platelets; weakly expressed by neutrophils and their precursors, more strongly expressed by monocytes and eosinophils than by neutrophils; more strongly expressed by lymphocytes than by neutrophils or monocytes; expression by macrophages is weak; expressed by osteoclasts; weakly expressed by CD34-positive stem cells; strongly expressed by mature B, T and NK lymphocytes; expressed by tonsillar plasma cells, peripheral blood plasma cells and reactive plasma cells produced in response to increased IL6 secretion, but weakly expressed if at all by normal bone marrow plasma cells; expressed by mast cells; there is no consensus as to whether follicular dendritic cells are positive or negative; different isoforms exist, formed by differential splicing of exons 4, 5 and 6 to give CD45RA (R = restricted), CD45RB and CD45RC respectively as well as CD45RO (lacking any expression of exons 4, 5

or 6); CD45 is the common epitope; CD45RA is expressed by plasmacytoid dendritic cells.

Expressed in T-ALL (almost all cases) and usually B-ALL but expression is not as strong as by mature T and B cells and about 20% of cases of B-ALL are negative; weakly expressed by blast cells of AML; strongly expressed in neoplasms of mature lymphocytes; expressed in NLPHL but not in classical Hodgkin lymphoma; sometimes expressed by myeloma cells but more often negative or weak.

Useful for gating on leucocytes of various lineages, often together with side scatter (SSC); used for gating for MRD evaluation and for MRD monitoring in B-ALL as it is often underexpressed in comparison with expression by haematogones; CD45RO is used in immunohistochemistry, with some MoAb having broad specificity for myeloid lineage as well as T cells and others being T-cell restricted (identifying antigen-experienced T cells).

CD47

An adhesion molecule, an inhibitory receptor expressed by virtually all cells including red cells and other myeloid cells, protecting against phagocytosis; binds to thrombospondin and SIRPα; a glycoprotein component of the Rh protein complex which links the Rh complex to protein 4.2 and band 3; important in neutrophil migration and activation in response to bacterial infection; mediates binding of platelets to thrombospondin of inflamed vascular endothelium; red cells of patients with hereditary spherocytosis resulting from lack of protein 4.2 lack CD47, and CD47 is also reduced in Rh^{NULL} cells; CD47 protects against autoimmune haemolytic anaemia by binding red cells to the inhibitory receptor, SIRPα, on macrophages; in aged erythrocytes a conformational change in CD47 leads to phagocytosis through SIRPα; downregulation of CD47 on haemopoietic cells leads to their engulfment by macrophages in HLH.

Expressed in CLL, NHL, multiple myeloma (80% of cases) and MGUS (39% of cases); mediates extranodal dissemination of NHL.

An anti-CD47 MoAb, magrolimab (hu5F9-G4, 5F9), synergises with rituximab to enhance phagocytosis of lymphoma cells by macrophages, and is undergoing trials in B-cell lymphomas; it is useful in AML and MDS; use of this MoAb interferes with ABO blood grouping.

CD49b

A membrane glycoprotein, α2 integrin; associates with CD29 to form $\alpha_2\beta_1$ integrin, platelet glycoprotein Ia/IIa (CD49b/CD29); expressed on megakaryocytes, platelets, B cells, activated T cells, monocytes, endothelial cells, fibroblasts and thymic epithelial cells.

Expression in CLL is prognostically very adverse.

Useful in the diagnosis of Glanzmann's thrombasthenia.

CD52

A GPI-anchored protein, expressed by thymocytes, T and B lymphocytes and NK cells, eosinophils, monocytes, macrophages and, to a lesser extent neutrophils; expressed by peripheral blood but not tissue dendritic cells; not expressed by normal Langerhans cells. Expressed in about a third of cases of T and NK cell lymphomas; expression in CLL is similar to expression by normal B cells; strongly expressed in a minority of cases of mantle cell lymphoma; can be expressed in MGUS, multiple myeloma and light-chain associated amyloidosis; expressed in Langerhans cell histiocytosis; expression is induced on the promyelocytes of acute promyelocytic leukaemia by exposure to all-*trans*-retinoic acid; expression is reduced in PNH. A MoAb, alemtuzumab, can result in long-term depletion of T lymphocytes when used *in vivo* and can be used for purging T lymphocytes *in vitro*; can be useful in T-PLL, mycosis fungoides and Sézary syndrome, and T-cell lymphomas; has been used in relapsed or refractory disease and for eliminating MRD in CLL (but use in CLL no longer advised); has been used for *in vivo* purging

for autologous stem cell transplantation in CLL; it may be useful in acquired bone marrow failure syndromes including aplastic anaemia, pure red cell aplasia and pure white cell aplasia; has a potential role in 'double hit' and 'double expresser' aggressive B-cell lymphomas, three quarters of which express CD52; may be useful in hairy cell variant leukaemia; has been used successfully for immune-related myocarditis induced by check-point inhibitors.

CD54

Intercellular adhesion molecule 1 (ICAM-1), expressed by activated B cells, activated T cells, plasma cells, dendritic cells, basophils, mast cells, macrophages, osteoclasts and activated endothelial cells including those of the bone marrow.

Expressed by the blast cells of about three quarters of cases of AML; sometimes expressed in CLL, by neoplastic mast cells, by myeloma cells and in some NHL.

CD55

A GPI-linked cell surface glycoprotein, decay-accelerating factor (DAF), binds complement components, C3b, C4b, C3bBb, C4b2a, disassembles C3/C5 convertase and protects against inappropriate complement activation; ligand for CD97; widely expressed including expression by erythroid cells, neutrophils, mast cells and plasma cells.

Reduced expression in PNH; CD55-deficient red cells have also been detected in a proportion of patients with lymphoproliferative disorders; red cell expression is reduced in hereditary spherocytosis. Expressed by neoplastic mast cells and plasma cells.

Useful in the diagnosis of PNH.

CD56

Neural cell adhesion molecule (N-CAM), a member of the immunoglobulin superfamily, expressed by NK cells (mature and immature but not pre-NK cells), a subset of CD4-positive T cells, a subset of CD8-positive T cells and a subset of plasmacytoid dendritic cells; expressed by activated lymphocytes; expressed by a subset (1–2%) of peripheral blood monocytes and a higher proportion in reactive monocytosis; may be expressed by neutrophils after G-CSF therapy; may be aberrantly expressed by granulocyte and monocyte precursors in regenerating bone marrow; expressed by bone marrow macrophages and osteoclasts; expressed by osteoblasts and endosteal lining cells; expressed by some non-haemopoietic cells; not expressed by normal plasma cells.

Usually expressed in large granular lymphocytic leukaemia of NK lineage and sometimes in large granular lymphocytic leukaemia of T lineage; expressed in blastic plasmacytoid dendritic cell neoplasm, aggressive NK-cell leukaemia/lymphoma and nasal-type NK-cell lymphoma; occasionally expressed in various types of cutaneous T-cell lymphoma; expressed in hepatosplenic T-cell lymphoma; expressed in 10–15% of cases of T-ALL in children particularly in cases of early T-cell precursor ALL, where expression occurs in approaching a third of cases in comparison with expression in about 5% of other cases of T-ALL; expressed in 10–15% of cases of AML; expression is seen in some cases of AML with minimal evidence of differentiation, AML with t(8;21), acute promyelocytic leukaemia (10–20% of cases), AML with monocytic differentiation, AML and transient abnormal myelopoiesis of Down's syndrome, therapy-related AML and AML with myelodysplasia-related changes; expression has been linked to a worse prognosis in AML in general and specifically in AML associated with t(8;21) and t(15;17); in AML with normal cytogenetics and lacking *FLT3* internal duplication, is indicative of a worse prognosis; expressed by monocytes in 80% of cases of CMML; expressed in many cases of multiple myeloma and, in one study, somewhat less often in plasma cell leukaemia; in another study, failure of expression in multiple

myeloma, seen in 20% of patients, was associated with worse survival; downregulated on extramedullary myeloma cells in comparison with bone marrow myeloma cells; expressed by plasma cells in less than 10% of cases of MGUS; rarely expressed in B-NHL; expressed in small cell carcinoma of the lung and neural-derived tumours such as neuroblastoma and astrocytoma – on flow cytometry, CD45-negativity with CD56-positivity can be used for the presumptive identification of these tumours; detection of CD45 negativity with CD56 and CD81 positivity has been recommended for the identification of circulating neuroblastoma cells; often expressed in rhabdomyosarcoma; in addition to tumours of neuroendocrine origin, is often expressed in adrenocortical and thyroid carcinomas; overall is expressed in about a quarter of carcinomas.

Important in the diagnosis of blastic plasmacytoid dendritic cell neoplasm; aberrant expression (with CD19) in AML suggests possible t(8;21); useful in the diagnosis of large granular lymphocytic leukaemia and NK-cell neoplasms; useful in MRD monitoring in AML; a CD45−, CD56+ immunophenotype on flow cytometry suggests a non-haemopoietic tumour such as a neuroendocrine tumour or rhabdomyosarcoma.

CD57

Expressed by NK cells, subsets of T cells including follicular helper T cells, B cells, monocytes and a subset of Schwann cells.

Lymphocytes of the autoimmune lymphoproliferative syndrome are CD3+, CD4−, CD8−, CD45RO− and CD57+; upregulated on T cells in viral infection and in primary HLH; usually expressed in large granular lymphocytic leukaemia of T lineage and sometimes in large granular lymphocytic leukaemia of NK lineage; expressed in angioimmunoblastic T-cell lymphoma; expressed in some carcinomas, for example, small cell carcinoma of the lung, and in neuroblastoma and Ewing's sarcoma.

Useful in the diagnosis of large granular lymphocytic leukaemia and NK-cell neoplasms.

CD58

Leucocyte function-associated antigen 3 (LFA-3), the ligand of CD2, occurs as a transmembrane protein with a cytoplasmic domain and as a GPI-anchored membrane protein; strongly expressed on leucocyte precursors, expression decreasing with maturation; expressed by dendritic cells, mast cells, erythrocytes, a proportion of lymphoid stem cells, endothelial cells, epithelial cells and fibroblasts; not expressed by normal plasma cells.

Expressed by blast cells in the majority of cases of AML and B-ALL; it is overexpressed in B-ALL in comparison with normal and regenerating B cells; expressed by myeloma cells and neoplastic mast cells.

Useful for MRD monitoring in B-ALL.

CD59

A GPI-linked cell surface glycoprotein, which associates with the final component of the complement pathway, C9, inhibiting incorporation of C5b-8 to form a membrane attack complex (hence 'protectin'); widely expressed including expression by erythrocytes, neutrophils, lymphocytes, monocytes, platelets, mast cells and plasma cells; has a signalling role in T-cell activation.

Expressed more strongly by neoplastic than normal mast cells; expressed in myeloma; reduced expression in PNH; CD59-deficient red cells have also been identified in a proportion of patients with lymphoproliferative disorders; a patient doubly heterozygous for different nonsense mutations in the *CD59* gene leading to CD59 deficiency was reported to have haemolytic anaemia and thrombosis causing cerebral infarction, but none of the other features of PNH; other patients of North African Jewish origin with a homozygous mutation had chronic haemolytic anaemia with exacerbations and relapsing polyneuropathy.

Useful in the diagnosis of PNH.

CD61

A surface membrane glycoprotein, the β3 integrin chain, GpIIIa; expressed by platelets and megakaryocytes (in association with CD41 forms GpIIb/IIIa, αIIbβ3 integrin, which is a receptor for fibrinogen, fibronectin, vitronectin and von Willebrand factor); expressed by monocytes, macrophages, osteoclasts and endothelial cells; expressed by mast cells.

Expressed by blast cells of acute megakaryoblastic leukaemia and may be expressed weakly by leukaemic cells of other subtypes of AML; megakaryocyte expression may be downregulated in MDS; expressed by neoplastic mast cells; expressed by some tumour cells, for example, melanoma and carcinoma of the breast, prostate and colon.

Used in some automated blood cell counters for an immunological platelet count; useful in the diagnosis of acute megakaryoblastic leukaemia and the diagnosis of Glanzmann's thrombasthenia (expression is reduced in most patients but some patients express a non-functional protein); useful for the immunohistochemical identification of megakaryocytes in MDS, MPN, MDS/MPN and acute panmyelosis with myelofibrosis; can be used in immunohistochemistry for the detection of platelet microthrombi, for example, in thrombotic thrombocytopenic purpura.

CD64

FcγRI – high affinity receptor for IgG1 and IgG3, expressed by CD34+/CD38+ progenitors, myeloblasts, promyelocytes, monoblasts, promonocytes, monocytes, macrophages and activated neutrophils and eosinophils (weak or negative on non-activated neutrophils), a subset of circulating myeloid dendritic cells, germinal centre dendritic cells; expression is up-regulated by interferon γ, G-CSF and IL10 and downregulated by IL4; upregulation on neutrophils is a sensitive indicator of infection or tissue injury with higher levels being more specific for sepsis.

CD64 expression has a high degree of both sensitivity and specificity for the diagnosis of AML with monocytic differentiation; also expressed, more weakly, in acute promyelocytic leukaemia.

Useful in the diagnosis of AML and for MRD monitoring.

CD65

Expressed by cells of neutrophil lineage from the promyelocyte stage onwards, by eosinophils and basophils, by a subset of monocytes and a subset of NK cells; a ligand for CD62E; expressed by some non-haemopoietic cells; CD65s is the sialylated form, which is expressed by granulocytes and monocytes.

CD65 is expressed by blast cells of many cases of AML; expression may be critical for extravascular infiltration by leukaemic cells; CD65s is also expressed by cells of AML, its expression appearing as CD34 expression disappears and before myeloperoxidase (MPO) expression; aberrantly expressed by cells of some cases of pro-B ALL, correlating with *KMT2A* rearrangement.

Useful for diagnosis and MRD monitoring in AML and for MRD monitoring in B-ALL.

CD66a–e

Members of the carcinoembryonic antigen family; GPI-linked; CD66b is expressed by neutrophils and metamyelocytes and weakly by myelocytes; expressed by epithelial cells; CD66c is expressed by promyelocytes and is downregulated on later cells; CD66e is expressed by neutrophils.

CD66c is sometimes expressed in AML; was expressed in 3/3 cases of AML with t(16;21) (p11;q22); aberrantly expressed in a subset of cases of B-ALL, particularly Ph-positive ALL (about 80%) and hyperdiploid ALL (about 60%); expressed in some carcinomas including colonic carcinoma.

Useful for MRD monitoring in B-ALL and in PNH diagnosis; CD66e is used for the detection of metastatic carcinoma in trephine biopsy sections.

CD68

Expressed by cells of neutrophil and monocyte lineage, plasmacytoid dendritic cells, osteoclasts and mast cells.

Expressed in AML and can be expressed weakly in B-ALL; expressed by melanoma cells.

Useful in immunohistochemistry for the recognition of myeloid differentiation and in the diagnosis of Langerhans cell histiocytosis.

CD68R

Expressed by cells of monocyte lineage including osteoclasts, and by plasmacytoid dendritic cells and mast cells.

Expressed by melanoma cells.

Useful for immunohistochemistry in AML for the detection of monocyte differentiation.

CD71

The transferrin receptor, expressed by early and late erythroid precursors and reticulocytes but not mature erythrocytes, by myeloblasts and promyelocytes, and by activated B and T lymphocytes and proliferating cells in general; more strongly expressed on erythroid cells than normal cells of other lineages; expressed by mast cells.

Expressed by immature erythroid cells in pure erythroid leukaemia; may be expressed in acute megakaryoblastic leukaemia; often expressed in T-ALL and may be expressed in B-ALL and aggressive lymphomas including ATLL, Burkitt lymphoma, Richter transformation of CLL, blastoid mantle cell lymphoma and some DLBCL; expressed by neoplastic mast cells; expressed by Reed–Sternberg cells; may be underexpressed in MDS.

Of some use in the diagnosis of pure erythroid leukaemia but not specific.

CD79a

Part of the immunoglobulin-associated heterodimeric B-cell antigen receptor complex; expressed by B cells and their precursors, and by plasma cells; although less specific than CD20, it is expressed both earlier and later in B-cell development and is expressed later than PAX5; MoAbs used for flow cytometry detect an intracellular epitope and therefore require permeabilisation of the cells; they are useful in determining B lineage; some MoAbs are positive with vascular smooth muscle and megakaryocytes.

Expressed by blast cells of B-ALL and in mature B-lineage leukaemias and lymphomas; expression in hairy cell leukaemia may be weak; expressed by neoplastic cells in NLPHL and expressed, more weakly, by the neoplastic cells of a significant minority of cases of classical Hodgkin lymphoma; can be aberrantly expressed by myeloblasts of AML, particularly AML associated with t(8;21), and also in T-ALL and T-NHL, by neoplastic erythroid cells and in blastic plasmacytoid dendritic cell neoplasm; myeloma cells are negative for CD79a in about 40% of cases, and expression is weak in another 15%.

Useful in the identification of B-lineage neoplasms and for MRD monitoring when aberrantly expressed in AML or T-ALL.

CD79b

Part of the B-cell antigen receptor complex, expressed by mature B cells and late B-cell precursors (pre-B cells); downregulated on B-cell activation.

Expressed in most neoplasms of mature B cells but weakly or not at all by the cells of CLL/SLL and in only about a half of cases of lymphoplasmacytoid lymphoma and a quarter of cases of hairy cell leukaemia; sometimes expressed in myeloma; expressed in cases of B-ALL.

An antibody–drug conjugate, polatuzumab vedotin, is useful in DLBCL and follicular lymphoma.

Weak or absent expression is useful in the diagnosis of CLL/SLL.

CD80

Expressed by T cells, activated B cells and some dendritic cells; expressed weakly by immature dendritic cells, such as those in skin and other peripheral tissues, but expressed strongly by mature dendritic cells in lymph nodes; expressed by monocytes.

Expressed in some cases of CLL and most cases of mantle cell lymphoma, follicular lymphoma, DLBCL and MZLs; expressed in the majority of cases of Langerhans cell histiocytosis.

Galiximab, a chimaeric human-monkey anti-CD80 MoAb, was under development for use in lymphoma but development was discontinued.

CD81

Broadly expressed by haemopoietic cells but not by erythrocytes, platelets or neutrophils; strongly expressed by B-cell precursors but downregulated on mature B cells; strongly expressed by plasma cells; expressed by immature dendritic cells, T lymphocytes, endothelial cells, epithelial cells and hepatocytes.

Compared with normal B-cell precursors, expression is weaker in three quarters of cases of B-ALL; more weakly expressed in CLL than by normal B cells; expression by myeloma cells may be weaker than expression by normal plasma cells; expression in myeloma is prognostically adverse; expressed by neuroblastoma cells.

Useful for MRD monitoring in B-ALL, CLL and myeloma.

CD86

Expressed by monocytes, B-cell precursors, activated B cells, memory B cells and germinal centre B cells; expressed weakly by immature dendritic cells, such as those in skin (Langerhans cells) and other peripheral tissues, but expressed strongly by mature dendritic cells in lymph nodes, for example, interdigitating reticulum cells.

Expressed by Hodgkin and Reed–Sternberg cells; expressed in some cases of AML including those with monocytic differentiation; often underexpressed in B-ALL in comparison with expression by normal B-cell precursors; expressed by neoplastic mast cells; expressed in about half of cases of multiple myeloma, expression correlating with a worse prognosis; usually expressed weakly or not at all by the cells of Langerhans cell histiocytosis.

Useful for MRD monitoring in B-ALL.

CD94

One of a group of killer inhibitory receptors that prevent cytotoxicity directed at autologous T cells; expressed by mature NK cells but not pre-NK cells or immature NK cells; expressed by a subset of T cells.

Expressed by cells of nasal-type T/NK lymphoma, aggressive NK-cell leukaemia/lymphoma and a minority of extranodal cytotoxic T-cell lymphomas but not cells of blastic NK-cell leukaemia/lymphoma.

CD99

Broadly expressed by many body cells, including expression by haemopoietic cells and strong expression by thymocytes but not expressed by normal T or B cells; erythrocytes are positive.

Overexpressed by the blast cells in the majority of cases of AML and ALL and expressed in a number of non-haemopoietic tumours; expressed in about 80% of cases of ALK-positive ALCL and in about 54% of ALK-negative cases; expressed in about 38% of DLBCL, expression correlating with advanced stage and non-germinal centre immunophenotype; expressed in Ewing's sarcoma and primitive neuroectodermal tumours (PNET).

Useful for MRD monitoring in T-ALL; used in immunohistochemistry for the identification of PNET/Ewing's sarcoma.

CD103

A cell surface antigen, αE integrin, which forms a heterodimer with β7 integrin; expressed by mucosa-associated T lymphocytes, other intra-epithelial T lymphocytes and a small subset of peripheral blood lymphocytes (2–6%); expressed by a subset of regulatory T cells in the gut and at sites of inflammation; expressed by monocytes.

Expressed in hairy cell leukaemia (but not in hairy cell leukaemia variant), in ATLL and in enteropathy-associated T-cell lymphoma and by lymphocytes of the closely related ulcerative jejunitis; expressed in some MZLs.

Useful in the diagnosis of hairy cell leukaemia and its differential diagnosis with hairy cell variant.

CD105

Endoglin, expressed by endothelial cells, activated monocytes, macrophages, early B-cell precursors, stromal cells of the bone marrow, proerythroblasts and some haemopoietic stem cells.

Expression is increased in erythroblasts in MDS and a combination of reduced CD71 expression and increased CD105 expression has reasonable sensitivity and specificity for distinguishing MDS from non-clonal cytopenia; expressed in a proportion of patients with AML, particularly in association with t(8;21) and bi-allelic *CEBPA* mutation; acute promyelocytic leukaemia has been variously reported to show consistent expression or consistent negativity; expressed in the majority of cases of B-ALL but less often in T-ALL.

Potentially useful in the diagnosis of MDS.

CD107a

A lysosomal membrane protein translocated to the cell surface on activation; expressed by activated platelets, activated cytotoxic T cells, activated NK cells, activated neutrophils and activated endothelial cells; necessary for efficient perforin delivery to lytic granules and for NK cell cytotoxicity.

Reduced expression by cytotoxic T cells and NK cells can be used to screen for familial HLH due to mutations in *UNC13D*, *STX11*, *STXBP2*, *RAB27A*, *LYST* and *AP3B1*.

CD110

Thrombopoietin receptor, expressed by a haemopoietic stem cell subset, megakaryocytes and, weakly, by platelets; expressed by common myeloid but not common lymphoid progenitor cells. Expressed in transient abnormal myelopoiesis of Down's syndromes and in *NPM1*-mutated AML.

CD116

The α chain of the receptor for granulocyte-macrophage colony-stimulating factor; expressed by monocytes, macrophages, neutrophils, eosinophils and dendritic cells; sometimes expressed by basophils but not by mast cells; expressed by some CD34-positive precursor cells and by promyelocytes, myelocytes and metamyelocytes; expressed by endothelial cells.

Expressed by some leukaemic blast cells, particularly in acute monoblastic/monocytic leukaemia; not expressed in ALL.

CD117

KIT, stem cell factor receptor, expressed by a proportion of haemopoietic precursors, myeloblasts, promyelocytes, megakaryoblasts, primitive erythroid cells, mast cells but not basophils, a subset of NK cells; expressed by early cells of neutrophil lineage but not those of eosinophil lineage; expressed by early B-lymphoid cells and immature thymic T cells; not expressed by plasma cells expressed by a range of non-haemopoietic cells.

Expressed by the blast cells of most cases of AML with megakaryoblasts as well as myeloblasts expressing the antigen; often negative in acute promyelocytic leukaemia and acute monoblastic leukaemia; expressed in systemic mastocytosis; expressed by plasma cells in about half of cases of MGUS and by about a third of cases of myeloma but usually not by the cells of plasma cell leukaemia; rarely expressed in T-ALL or mixed phenotype acute leukaemia in which cells correspond to a very early multipotent (T/myeloid) thymocyte; expressed in early T-cell precursor ALL; possibly expressed in ALCL (studies conflict), expressed in some non-haemopoietic tumours.

Useful in the diagnosis and for MRD monitoring of AML and in the diagnosis of systemic mastocytosis.

CD123

The interleukin 3 receptor α chain, IL3Rα, variably expressed by haemopoietic stem cells, eosinophils, monocytes, megakaryocytes, B lymphocytes and endothelial cells but not T lymphocytes or neutrophils; expressed by plasmacytoid but not myeloid dendritic cells; expressed by basophils but not normal or reactive mast cells; dendritic cells and basophils are both strongly CD123 positive but basophils are HLA-DR negative whereas dendritic cells are HLA-DR positive.

Expressed by blast cells of the majority of cases of AML but not expressed by normal CD34-positive, CD38-negative bone marrow stem cells; expressed by leukaemic stem cells in AML; expression in AML correlates with poor prognosis although it is usually positive in the good prognosis category associated with *NPM1* mutation; aberrantly expressed in a quarter to two thirds of mast cell neoplasms; expressed, together with CD4 and CD56, in blastic plasmacytoid dendritic cell neoplasm; expressed by bone marrow plasmacytoid dendritic cells in CMML; not expressed by normal lymphoid progenitors but expressed by blast cells in about 90% of cases of B-ALL and in about 40% of cases of T-ALL; in B-ALL, associated with high hyperdiploidy; often overexpressed in B-ALL in comparison with expression by haematogones; moderately to strongly expressed in hairy cell leukaemia

(95% of cases), in some atypical cases of CLL – in which condition it correlates with CD11c expression – and in some transformed chronic lymphoproliferative disorders; much less often expressed in hairy cell leukaemia variant (9%) and splenic lymphoma with villous lymphocytes/splenic MZL (3%); not usually expressed in follicular lymphoma or mantle cell lymphoma; expressed by Hodgkin/Reed–Sternberg cells in about 60% of cases of classical Hodgkin lymphoma.

Monoclonal antibodies (including flotetuzumab) and CAR T cells for therapeutic use in AML and blastic plasmacytoid dendritic cell neoplasm are under development; a bispecific CD3-CD123 MoAb also has potential in blastic plasmacytoid dendritic cell neoplasm and tagraxofusp, a CD123-directed cytotoxin, has been shown to be effective.

Useful for MRD monitoring in B-ALL and AML and in the diagnosis of hairy cell leukaemia and blastic plasmacytoid dendritic cell neoplasm.

CD127

The interleukin 7 receptor α chain (IL7Rα), which combines with the β chain, CD132, to form a high affinity receptor, IL7R; expressed by most T cells, being downregulated on T-cell activation; expressed by B-cell precursors and monocytes.

Downregulated in primary HLH.
Can be used in the diagnosis of HLH.

CD133

Expressed by stem cell/progenitor cell subsets that can give rise to endothelial cells as well as haemopoietic cells and B lymphocytes; expressed by some CD34-positive B-lymphocyte precursors.

Expressed by blast cells of the majority of cases of AML and ALL; expressed by leukaemic stem cells; in patients with AML, expression correlates with other markers of immaturity with acute promyelocytic leukaemia not showing expression; expression is more frequent in B-ALL than T-ALL and is characteristic of B-ALL with t(4;11) and rearrangement of the *KMT2A* gene; expressed by some non-haemopoietic tumours.

CD135

FLT3, a receptor tyrosine kinase encoded by *FLT3*; expressed by multipotent stem cells, myelomonocytic precursors and early B-cell progenitors.

Expressed by blast cells in ALL, AML and the blast crisis of CML and in a subset of acute mixed phenotypic T-myeloid leukaemia.

CAR T cells for use in AML are under development.

CD138

Heparan sulphate proteoglycan, an adhesion molecule, LFA-3 or Syndecan-1 (syndecan, from the Greek = stick together); expressed by pre-B cells and late post-germinal centre B cells but not circulating or germinal centre B cells; expressed by plasma cells including early plasma cells but not expressed by reactive plasmablasts; may be expressed by myeloblasts; expressed by epithelial cells.

Expressed by myeloma cells; expressed in some lymphomas including lymphoplasmacytic lymphoma and some cases of DLBCL, including plasmablastic lymphoma; CLL cells show weak or moderate cytoplasmic and membrane expression; expressed in HIV-associated primary effusion lymphoma; reported to be expressed in 50–90% of cases of carcinoma; rarely expressed in mesothelioma and, since most carcinomas that metastasise to the pleura do express CD138, this can be useful in differential diagnosis; expressed in 50% of melanomas; expressed in a half of osteosarcomas and in a larger proportion of osteoblastomas; occasionally expressed in soft tissue tumours.

CD138 is being investigated as a target of CAR T cells in multiple myeloma.

Useful for diagnosis and MRD monitoring in myeloma.

CD157

A GPI-anchored protein with structural similarities to CD38; expressed by myeloid precursors, neutrophils, monocytes, mast cells, macrophages, follicular dendritic cells, endothelial cells, bone marrow stromal cells, gut epithelial cells, mesothelial cells and α and β cells of the pancreas; an important mediator of neutrophil adhesion and migration.

Can be used in the diagnosis of PNH.

CD158a–k

NK cell receptors; members of the KIR (killer inhibitory receptor) family and immunoglobulin gene superfamily; expressed by a NK subset and a smaller proportion of T cells; following engagement of CD158a, inhibition of NK cell activity is seen, preventing cytotoxicity directed at autologous HLA-I-positive cells.

In T-cell large granular lymphocytic and NK-cell leukaemias, there may be failure to express any CD158 antigens or there may be expression of only one of CD158a, CD158b and CD158e; abnormal expression patterns are of particular value in the diagnosis of NK cell neoplasms since there is no readily available marker of monoclonality for this lineage; in γδ hepatosplenic T-cell lymphoma, there may be aberrant expression of two or three of CD158 a, b and e; CD158k is often expressed in Sézary syndrome and mycosis fungoides and is less often expressed in other cutaneous T-cell lymphomas and is a possible target for immunotherapy.

Useful as a surrogate marker for clonality in NK cell neoplasms.

CD160

A GPI-linked or transmembrane protein, a costimulatory molecule, expressed by 20% of CD8+ αβ+ T cells, by γδ T cells and by CD56 weak/CD16+ highly cytolytic NK cells.

Aberrantly expressed in hairy cell leukaemia and CLL.

Useful for MRD monitoring in CLL.

CD161

One of a group of killer inhibitory receptors that prevent cytotoxicity directed at autologous T cells; expressed by most NK cells, both mature and immature, pre-NK cells, a subset of T cells, a subset of thymocytes and by follicular dendritic cells; CD161++CD8+ T cells are a tissue-infiltrating population secreting cytokines that are important for mucosal immunity.

CD161 is expressed in aggressive and nasal type NK-cell leukaemia/lymphoma but not blastic NK-cell leukaemia /lymphoma; often expressed in T-PLL.

CD163

A scavenger receptor for haemoglobin, binding to haemoglobin–haptoglobin complexes and to free haemoglobin in plasma, expressed by macrophages and weakly by circulating monocytes (expression being upregulated by activation during infection and in MPN); mediates the interaction between macrophages and erythroblasts; macrophage expression is upregulated by corticosteroids, interferon gamma, IL6 and IL10; IL4 greatly reduces expression; not expressed by osteoclasts; CD163 expression, detected by immunocytochemistry, is very specific for the detection of macrophages.

CD163 may be expressed in AML with monocytic differentiation but is not sufficiently sensitive for the detection of myeloid sarcoma or leukaemias of monocyte lineage; not expressed by neoplastic cells in Langerhans cell histiocytosis.

Immunohistochemical demonstration of CD163 expression can be useful for highlighting macrophages and for demonstrating the monocytic component in CMML and atypical chronic myeloid leukaemia.

CD180

Expressed by mantle and marginal zone B cells, monocytes and dendritic cells.

Expressed in about 60% of cases of CLL but expression is weaker than that of normal B cells; expression is significantly stronger in those with hypermutated *IGVH* genes than in those without, but is still less than in normal B cells; expression is stronger in splenic diffuse red pulp small B-cell lymphoma than in other lymphoproliferative disorders.

CD200

Member of the immunoglobulin superfamily; expressed by thymocytes, B cells, a subset of T cells (follicular helper T cells), dendritic cells, neurons and endothelial cells; not expressed by NK cells or normal plasma cells.

Expressed in 95% of B-ALL; T-ALL is negative; may be expressed in AML, particularly in AML associated with t(8;21) or inv(16); expressed by myeloma cells in two thirds to three quarters of cases, lack of expression correlating with worse prognosis in one study but not in another; strongly expressed in CLL and hairy cell leukaemia in comparison with normal B cells and the cells of most other lymphoproliferative disorders; expressed less strongly in splenic MZL and usually weak or negative in mantle cell lymphoma, follicular lymphoma and splenic diffuse red pulp small B-cell lymphoma; usually expressed in neuroendocrine tumours.

Useful in CLL diagnosis and in differentiating CLL from other CD5+ lymphoproliferative disorders; useful in MRD monitoring in B-ALL as about half of cases show overexpression or underexpression in comparison with normal B-cell precursors; has potential for MRD monitoring in multiple myeloma.

CD203c

Expressed by basophils and mast cells.
Useful in the diagnosis of acute basophilic leukaemia.

CD207

Langerin, a lectin expressed on immature Langerhans cells.
Expressed in Langerhans cell histiocytosis.

Immunohistochemistry for CD207 is important for the diagnosis of Langerhans cell histiocytosis.

CD227

Epithelial membrane antigen, MUC1, expressed by epithelial cells, plasma cells, early erythroid cells and monocytes.

Expressed in ALCL (more often in ALK-positive than ALK-negative cases) and primary effusion lymphoma; expressed by the neoplastic cells of NLPHL; may be expressed in myeloma; expressed in acute monocytic/monoblastic leukaemia and in some erythroleukaemias; many carcinomas are positive.

Used in immunohistochemistry.

CD229

Expressed by T cells, B cells and plasma cells; overexpressed by myeloma cells and their clonogenic precursors; expressed in MGUS.

CD235a

Glycophorin A, expressed by erythroid cells, expressed later than glycophorin C by erythroid precursors and later than CD71.

Useful in the diagnosis of pure erythroid leukaemia.

Applicable to immunohistochemistry for the diagnosis of pure erythroid leukaemia.

CD235b

Glycophorin B, expressed by erythroid cells.
Useful in the diagnosis of pure erythroid leukaemia.

CD236

Glycophorin D, expressed by a stem cell subset and by erythroblasts.

CD236R

Glycophorin C, expressed by a stem cell subset and by erythroblasts; expressed earlier than glycophorin A.

The MoAb, ret40f, is suitable for immuno-histochemistry.

CD241

Rh-associated glycoprotein, expressed by erythroid cells, deficiency leads to the Rh null phenotype.

CD246

ALK protein, absent from all post-natal tissues except rare cells in the brain. Expressed in T-lineage ALK-positive ALCL and in ALK-positive large B-cell lymphoma; expressed by some non-haemopoietic tumours. Essential in immunohistochemistry for the diagnosis of ALK-positive ALCL and ALK-positive large B-cell lymphoma.

CD269

Expressed by myeloma cells and can be the target of CAR T cell therapy.

CD274

Programmed cell death ligand 1, PD-L1.

Expressed in AML, sometimes in DLBCL and in many solid tumours; high expression in AML has been found to correlate with unfavourable recurrent mutations but not necessarily with a worse prognosis; strong expression, seen in about half of patients with peripheral T-cell lymphoma, correlates with worse survival.

Avelumab is an anti-PD-L1 MoAb leading to up-regulation of the immune response; of potential use in AML and classical (but not nodular lymphocyte predominant) Hodgkin lymphoma; durvalumab and atezolizumab are used in non-haematological neoplasms and are of potential value in myeloma.

CD279

Programmed cell death protein 1, PD-1, expressed by some B cells, activated T cells including follicular helper T cells, and macrophages; binding of PD-1 of T cells to PD-L1 (CD274) leads to T cell inhibition.

Expressed in T-cell lymphomas of follicular helper T-cell phenotype such as angioimmunoblastic T-cell lymphoma; expressed in Sézary syndrome; may be expressed in cutaneous T-cell lymphoma, peripheral T-cell lymphoma, not otherwise specified and T-cell large granular lymphocytic leukaemia; expressed in Richter syndrome but not in DLBCL or CLL. The monoclonal antibody, pidilizumab, is of potential value in myeloma; MoAbs, nivolumab and pembrolizumab, have potential for the treatment of CLL, classical Hodgkin lymphoma and primary mediastinal B-cell lymphoma, but the initial results of nivolumab in DLBCL were disappointing; nivolumab plus ibrutinib may have an advantage in Richter syndrome, but overall the efficacy of nivolumab and pembrolizumab in Richter syndrome is poor; nivolumab plus ibrutinib appears to be no better than ibrutinib alone in CLL, follicular lymphoma and DLBCL; nivolumab can be effective in EBV-associated HLH; pembrolizumab may be efficacious in extranodal NK/T-cell lymphoma, nasal type; camrelizumab may be of benefit in Hodgkin lymphoma; cemiplimab is used in non-haematological neoplasms.

Used in immunohistochemistry.

CD300e

Expressed by monocytes and myeloid dendritic cells.

CD303

Expressed by plasmacytoid dendritic cells.

Expressed in blastic plasmacytoid dendritic cell neoplasm.

Useful in the diagnosis of blastic plasmacytoid dendritic cell neoplasm.

CD304

Neuropilin 1, expressed by B-lymphoid progenitors, normal erythroid progenitors, plasmacytoid dendritic cells and plasma cells.

Expressed in about a quarter of cases of AML; expressed in blastic plasmacytoid dendritic cell neoplasm; expressed in 40% of cases of B-ALL.

Useful in the diagnosis of blastic plasmacytoid dendritic cell neoplasm; can be used for MRD monitoring in B-ALL as it is often over-expressed in comparison with expression on haematogones.

CD305

An inhibitor of B-cell receptor antigen signalling.

Strongly expressed in hairy cell leukaemia; more strongly expressed in mantle cell lymphoma than follicular lymphoma; expressed in about two thirds of cases of CLL, expression being associated with a better prognosis.

CD319

SLAM7, expressed by normal plasma cells, not expressed by B cells unless activated; expressed by NK cells, CD8+ T cells and mature dendritic cells.

Expressed in monoclonal gammopathy of undetermined significance, in multiple myeloma, in Waldenström's macroglobulinaemia and in plasmablastic lymphoma; overexpressed by monocytes in myeloproliferative neoplasms with *JAK2* V617F.

Elotuzumab, a humanised MoAb directed against CD319, is of use in myeloma, when combined with lenalidomide and dexamethasone, and of potential value in myelofibrosis.

CD324

E-cadherin; expressed by cells of epithelial origin; expressed by erythroblasts, from early pro-erythroblasts onwards, so detects earlier cells than anti-glycophorin antibodies. Useful in immunohistochemistry, particularly for the identification of pure erythroid leukaemia.

CD326

Ep-CAM, expressed by epithelial cells. Can be used in flow cytometry to identify cells of epithelial origin in carcinocythaemia.

CD335

Expressed by NK cells. Expressed in about 90% of NK cell neoplasms; aberrantly expressed in about a fifth of T-cell lymphomas, particularly T-cell large granular lymphocytic leukaemia, mycosis fungoides and ALK+ ALCL. Used in MRD monitoring in T-ALL.

CD340

HER2, human epidermal growth factor receptor 2. Expressed by some breast cancers and other cancers. Immunohistochemistry is relevant in carcinoma since expression is indicative of a likely response to trastuzumab, directed at this antigen; preferably done on the primary tumour rather than on bone marrow metastases when tissue of the primary tumour is available.

Antibodies without CD numbers

κ

Immunoglobulin light chain, expressed, together with a heavy chain, on the surface membrane of about two-thirds of B cells and within the cytoplasm of a similar proportion of plasma cells; polyclonal antisera are preferred. Very important in demonstrating clonality in B-lineage neoplasms. Widely used in immunohistochemistry but the detection of κ or λ mRNA by *in situ* hybridisation is an alternative technique.

λ

Immunoglobulin light chain, expressed, together with a heavy chain, on the surface membrane of about a third of B cells and within the cytoplasm of a similar proportion of plasma cells. Very important in demonstrating clonality in B-lineage neoplasms. Widely used in immunohistochemistry but the detection of κ or λ mRNA by *in situ* hybridisation is an alternative technique.

γ

Heavy chain of IgG; expressed, together with a light chain, on the surface membrane of B cells and within the cytoplasm of plasma cells; polyclonal antisera are preferred.

α

Heavy chain of IgA; expressed, together with a light chain, on the surface membrane of B cells and within the cytoplasm of plasma cells; polyclonal antisera are preferred.

μ

Heavy chain of IgM; expressed within the cytoplasm of pre-B cells and, together with a light chain, on the surface membrane of B cells; expressed within the cytoplasm of plasma cells; polyclonal antisera are preferred.

δ

Heavy chain of IgD; expressed, together with a light chain, on the surface membrane of B cells and within the cytoplasm of plasma cells; polyclonal antisera are preferred.

ε

Heavy chain of IgE; expressed, together with a light chain, on the surface membrane of B cells and within the cytoplasm of plasma cells; polyclonal antisera are preferred.

7.1

See NG2.

ALK1

See CD246.

annexin A1

Expressed by neutrophils, monocytes, macrophages and myeloid precursors. Has a high degree of sensitivity and specificity for hairy cell leukaemia, among B-cell neoplasms; not expressed in splenic MZL or hairy cell variant leukaemia.

basogranulin

Expressed by basophils. Used in immunohistochemistry.

BCL2

A widely expressed anti-apoptotic protein; expressed by T cells, B cells, NK cells, CD34-positive haemopoietic stem cells, myeloblasts, promyelocytes, myelocytes, monocytes and mast cells; not expressed by normal plasmacytoid dendritic cells. Expressed in proliferation centres in CLL and in neoplastic follicles in follicular lymphoma but not in reactive follicular hyperplasia; often expressed in NHL; often expressed in classical Hodgkin lymphoma; expressed in blastic plasmacytoid dendritic cell neoplasm. A BCL2 inhibitor, venetoclax, is potentially useful in a wide range of haematological neoplasms including CLL, follicular lymphoma, mantle cell lymphoma, multiple myeloma, AML, ALL, blastic plasmacytoid dendritic cell neoplasm and potentially high grade B-cell lymphoma with *BCL2* and *MYC* rearrangement. Detection of expression by immunohistochemistry is important in the diagnosis of follicular lymphoma; expression can also be detected by flow cytometry after permeabilisation; co-expression of BCL2 and MYC is prognostically adverse in DLBCL.

BCL6

Expressed by normal germinal centre B cells. Expressed in lymphomas of germinal centre origin (Burkitt lymphoma, follicular lymphoma and some DLBCL), in B-ALL with t(1;19)(q23;p13.3), in some ALCL, T-ALL and by neoplastic cells of NLPHL but not usually those of classical Hodgkin lymphoma; not expressed in mantle cell lymphoma. Used in immunohistochemistry.

BCL10

Nuclear expression in some extranodal MZLs of MALT type.

BOB.1

Expressed by normal B cells. Expressed in most B-NHL; expressed in NLPHL but negative or weak/focal in classical Hodgkin lymphoma.

BRAF^{V600E}

An aberrant protein expressed when there is a V600E mutation in the *BRAF* gene; not expressed in normal cells. Expressed in hairy cell leukaemia, Langerhans cell histiocytosis, Erdheim–Chester disease, Rosai–Dorfman disease and melanoma when the V600E mutation is present. Vemurafenib, a MoAb directed at V600E-mutated BRAF, is effective in hairy cell leukaemia, Langerhans cell histiocytosis and Erdheim–Chester disease; dabrafenib is similarly targeted at mutant BRAF and is effective in Langerhans cell histiocytosis and Rosai–Dorfman disease. Useful in the diagnosis and for MRD monitoring in hairy cell leukaemia with a *BRAF*^{V600E} mutation; useful in the diagnosis of Langerhans cell histiocytosis and metastatic melanoma.

calprotectin

Expressed by late neutrophil precursors and monocytes, previously known as calgranulin. Used in immunohistochemistry.

carcinoembryonic antigen

CD66e; *see* CD66a–e.

chromogranin

Used in immunochemistry for the identification of neuroendocrine carcinomas.

cyclin D1

A cyclin encoded by *CCND1*; widely expressed in human tissues with the strength of nuclear expression varying during the cell cycle. Nuclear expression occurs in 95% of cases of mantle cell lymphoma, in hairy cell leukaemia (more weakly) and in about 16% of cases of myeloma (strong in about 20% of patients with t(11;14), weaker in another 30%); expressed in proliferation centres in CLL/SLL. Important in the diagnosis of mantle cell lymphoma.

cytokeratin

Expressed by epithelial cells. Various cytokeratins are expressed by tumours of epithelial origin, including thymomas. Applicable to flow cytometry but mainly used in immunohistochemistry; there are broad spectrum and narrow spectrum MoAbs; immunohistochemistry with CK7 and CK20 narrow spectrum MoAbs is useful in indicating the tissue of origin when there are bone marrow metastases of carcinoma; broad spectrum MoAb are sometimes positive in ALCL and plasma cell neoplasms.

DBA.44

Appears **not** to have the CD72 specificity that was previously reported; expressed by B cells and some macrophages. Expressed in hairy cell leukaemia. Useful in immunohistochemistry for the diagnosis of hairy cell leukaemia.

desmin

Expressed in muscle cells. Used in immunohistochemistry for the identification of rhabdomyosarcoma.

E-cadherin

See CD324.

eosinophil major basic protein

Expressed by cells of eosinophil lineage. Used in immunohistochemistry.

eosinophil peroxidase

Expressed by cells of eosinophil lineage. Used in immunohistochemistry.

Ep-CAM

See CD326.

epithelial membrane antigen

See CD227.

ERG

Expressed in the nuclei of endothelial cells. Expressed in vascular tumours and lymphangiomas, some prostatic carcinomas and myeloid sarcomas.

FLI1

Expressed in the nuclei of endothelial cells. Expressed in tumours of endothelial origin, Ewing's sarcoma (90% of cases), PNET and ALL.

fluorescent aerolysin (FLAER)

Not an antibody but binds to GPI. Very useful in the diagnosis of PNH.

FMC7

The widely used MoAb, FMC7, which appears to bind to a particular cholesterol-dependent conformation of an epitope of CD20, probably a multimeric CD20 complex; expressed by mature B cells. Expressed in B-lineage NHL and hairy cell leukaemia but not in CLL. Useful in the diagnosis of CLL.

glycophorin

See CD235a, CD235b, CD236, CD236R.

granzyme

A family of cytotoxic lymphocyte proteins, granzyme A, B and M, expressed in the cytoplasm of NK cells, cytotoxic T cells and neutrophils; granzyme B is expressed by plasmacytoid dendritic cells. Expressed by aggressive NK-cell lymphoma, subcutaneous panniculitis-like T-cell lymphoma, enteropathy-type T-cell lymphoma and nasal-type extranodal T/NK-cell lymphoma. Used in immunohistochemistry but not often in flow cytometry as it is a cytoplasmic antigen.

HER2

See CD340.

HHV8-LANA1

Human herpesvirus 8 latency-associated nuclear antigen 1. Expressed in primary effusion lymphoma.

HLA-DR

Human leucocyte antigen-DR, expressed by haemopoietic stem cells and myeloblasts but not promyelocytes or more mature cells of granulocyte lineage, expressed by cells of monocyte lineage including macrophages, expressed by B-lineage lymphoid cells at all stages of maturation; expressed by activated T cells, for example, in viral infections, but not by most normal mature T cells; expressed by NK cells and plasmacytoid and myeloid dendritic cells; not expressed by normal plasma cells. Upregulated on T cells in viral infection; upregulation on T cells is useful in the diagnosis of HLH; expressed by blast cells in B-ALL, the majority of cases of AML and 10−20% of cases of T-ALL; expressed in mature B-cell neoplasms and in some cases of multiple myeloma and plasma cell leukaemia; not usually expressed in acute promyelocytic leukaemia or AML with *NPM1* rearrangement; strongly expressed in blastic plasmacytoid dendritic cell neoplasm. A CD34-negative, HLA-DR-negative, CD11b-negative immunophenotype is useful in the diagnosis of acute promyelocytic leukaemia; CD34-negative, HLA-DR-negative can also be indicative of AML with *NPM1* mutation.

immunoglobulin

Antibody molecules, each composed of two identical heavy chains and two identical light chains; expressed on the surface membrane of B cells (SmIg) and within the cytoplasm of plasma cells (cIg); the order of expression with maturation within the B lineage is: cμ chain (pre-B cell); Sm IgM; SmIgD; Sm IgG, IgA or IgE; cIg (plasma cell). Expressed in pre-B ALL (cμ), mature B-cell neoplasms (SmIg) and within the cytoplasm in myeloma and plasma cell leukaemia (cIg); lymphoplasmacytic lymphoma expresses both cIg and SmIg. Provides important evidence of clonality since Ig of neoplastic cells has either κ or λ light chain but not both; more weakly expressed in CLL than in other mature B-lineage neoplasms. *See also* κ, λ, γ, α, μ, ε, δ.

Ki-67

A proliferation marker, expressed in the nuclei of proliferating haemopoietic and lymphoid cells. Expressed in high-grade lymphomas. Useful in immunohistochemistry, using the MoAb MIB1, for assessing the aggressiveness of a lymphoma; useful in the diagnosis of Burkitt lymphoma, in which the great majority of neoplastic cells are positive; correlates with prognosis in follicular lymphoma and mantle cell lymphoma.

KIT

See CD117.

LEF1

Lymphoid enhancer-binding factor 1, expressed in the nucleus of T cells and pro-B cells but not mature B cells. Expressed in the nucleus of CLL cells but not other small B-cell neoplasms; sometimes expressed in DLBCL.

LMP1

Latent membrane protein 1, an EBV-encoded protein that can be detected immunohistochemically in many but not all lymphomas that carry EBV; in some cases *in situ* hybridisation is necessary to identify EBV in lymphoma cells. A potential target of T-cell therapy in EBV-related B and T/NK cell lymphomas.

lysozyme

Expressed within the cytoplasm of cells of neutrophil and monocyte lineage. Used in immunohistochemistry.

mast cell tryptase

An enzyme expressed by normal mast cells; not expressed by normal basophils. Expressed by neoplastic mast cells; neoplastic basophils in CML, primary myelofibrosis, MDS, and acute and chronic basophilic leukaemia may express mast cell tryptase; expression by basophils is generally weaker than that of mast cells; blast cells of AML may be positive. Detection of expression by immunohistochemistry is important in the diagnosis of systemic mastocytosis.

melanA

Expressed in melanoma.

MNDA

Myeloid cell nuclear differentiation antigen, expressed by myeloid cells and B lymphocytes; a polyclonal antiserum is available. Often expressed in nodal MZL and extranodal MZL; expressed in about a quarter of cases of splenic MZL and lymphoplasmacytic lymphoma but usually negative in mantle cell lymphoma, CLL, follicular lymphoma and DLBCL.

MUM1/IRF4

Multiple myeloma oncogene 1/interferon regulatory factor 4; expressed by late germinal centre and post-germinal centre somatically hypermutated B cells, plasma cells and a small proportion of T cells (activated T cells). Expressed in multiple myeloma, lymphoplasmacytic lymphoma, classical Hodgkin lymphoma (but weak or negative in NLPHL), primary effusion lymphoma and DLBCL with a non-germinal-centre phenotype; strongly expressed in large B-cell lymphoma with *IRF4* rearrangement; expression is reported in 40–90% of cases of CLL/SLL, without any correlation with mutational status; expressed in some cases of ATLL and ALCL. Useful in the histological diagnosis of B-lineage neoplasms; can also be expressed in ALCL, angioimmunoblastic T-cell lymphoma, ATLL and other T-cell lymphomas; expressed in melanoma.

MYC

Expressed by some germinal centre B cells. Expressed in Burkitt lymphoma and about a third of DLBCL. Co-expression of BCL2 and MYC is prognostically adverse in DLBCL.

myeloperoxidase (MPO)

Expressed in the primary granules of cells of neutrophil and eosinophil lineage from the late myeloblast stage onwards; more weakly expressed by monocytes; can be detected cytochemically, as well as by flow cytometric immunophenotyping after cell permeabilisation. Expressed by the blast cells of the majority of cases of AML and, by definition, by the blast cells of mixed phenotype acute leukaemia; weakly expressed in some B-ALL with an otherwise typical B-ALL phenotype. Useful for diagnosis and MRD monitoring of AML; essential for the diagnosis of mixed phenotype acute leukaemia.

myoglobin

Expressed by muscle cells. Used in immunohistochemistry for the identification of rhabdomyosarcoma.

neutrophil elastase

Expressed by promyelocytes and myelocytes but weak or negative in more mature cells. Used in immunohistochemistry.

NG2

Neuroglial 2 antigen, chondroitin sulphate; monoclonal antibody 7.1; expressed on CD34+CD38+ haemopoietic precursors. Expressed in *KMT2A* (*MLL*)-rearranged ALL and AML with monocytic differentiation. Useful for MRD monitoring in B-ALL and AML.

NPM1

Normally ubiquitously expressed in the nucleus. Expression in the cytoplasm as well as the nucleus is a surrogate marker for *NPM1* mutation in AML.

OCT-2

Expressed by normal B cells. Expressed in most B-NHL; expressed in NLPHL but negative, weak or focal in classical Hodgkin lymphoma.

PAX5

A B-cell transcription factor; expressed in the nucleus from pro-B cells onwards but not expressed by plasma cells. Expressed in B-ALL, CLL, B-lineage NHL, hairy cell leukaemia and in Hodgkin and Reed–Sternberg cells of classical Hodgkin lymphoma but expression may be weak; expressed in NLPHL; in some B-ALL is expressed only weakly; expressed in a minority of cases of multiple myeloma, expression correlating with expression of CD20 and cyclin D1; may be aberrantly expressed in AML associated with t(8;21); may be expressed by neuroendocrine tumours. Useful in the histological diagnosis of B-lineage neoplasms.

perforin

A cytotoxic lymphocyte protein, expressed by NK cells and cytotoxic CD8-positive T cells (γδ T cells and a subset of αβ T cells); is inserted into the membrane of a target cell, creating a pore through which cytotoxic enzymes, granzymes, can enter with the resultant activation of caspases leading to apoptosis; expressed by few cells in normal bone marrow. Expressed by aggressive NK-cell lymphoma, subcutaneous panniculitis-like T-cell lymphoma, enteropathy-type T-cell lymphoma and nasal-type extranodal T/NK-cell lymphoma. Used in immunohistochemistry but not often in flow cytometry as it is a cytoplasmic antigen; used in the diagnosis of primary HLH, in which it is upregulated on CD4-positive T cells; useful in the diagnosis of T-cell large granular lymphocytic leukaemia and other T/NK-cell lymphomas.

programmed cell protein 1

See CD279.

programmed cell death ligand 1

See CD274.

prostate-specific antigen

Used in immunohistochemistry for the diagnosis of prostatic cancer.

prostatic acid phosphatase

Used in immunohistochemistry for the diagnosis of prostatic cancer.

ROR1

Expressed by B-cell progenitors but not mature B cells or T cells. Expressed in CLL and in less than 10% of cases of B-ALL; also expressed in mantle cell lymphoma and more weakly, in MZL. Cirmtuzumab vedotin is an antibody–drug conjugate of potential value in CLL and other B-lineage neoplasms. Possibly useful in the differential diagnosis of CD5-positive B-lineage neoplasms.

rough endoplasmic reticulum-associated antigen

Identified with monoclonal antibody VS38c; expressed by plasma cells, osteoblasts and some bone marrow stromal cells. Expressed in multiple myeloma and in some cases of non-haemopoietic tumours including some soft tissue sarcomas, osteosarcomas, carcinomas and melanomas. Used in immunohistochemistry as a sensitive but not specific marker of plasma cells and plasma cell neoplasms.

S100

Expressed by chondrocytes, adipocytes, myoepithelial cells, macrophages, Langerhans cells, dendritic cells, Schwann cells, keratinocytes and melanocytes. Expressed in Langerhans cell histiocytosis, in melanoma, in certain tumours of neural origin and in some carcinomas. Used in immunohistochemistry for the identification of melanoma and certain other tumours; expressed in neuroendocrine carcinomas; 20% of breast cancers are positive.

SOX11

Normally expressed in the central nervous system, expression being nuclear. Positive in the majority of cases of mantle cell lymphoma but negative in leukaemic, non-nodal cases with mutated *IGVH* genes; useful in cases in which cyclin D1 staining is equivocal; may be expressed in hairy cell leukaemia; expressed in lymphoblastic leukaemia/lymphoma and about half of cases of Burkitt lymphoma.

synaptophysin

Used in immunochemistry for the identification of neuroendocrine carcinomas.

tartrate-resistant acid phosphatase

Expressed by osteoclasts, mast cells, Langerhans cells and macrophages. Expressed in hairy cell leukaemia. Useful in the diagnosis of hairy cell leukaemia.

T-cell receptor (TCR) αβ

A surface membrane receptor expressed by the majority of circulating T cells. Expressed by some cases of T-ALL and the majority of cases of mature T-lineage neoplasms.

T-cell receptor (TCR) γδ

A surface membrane receptor expressed by a small minority of circulating T cells. Sometimes expressed in T-ALL but less often than TCRαβ; usually expressed in hepatosplenic T-cell lymphoma. Important in the diagnosis of hepatosplenic T-cell lymphoma.

terminal deoxynucleotidyl transferase (TdT)

A DNA polymerase that catalyses terminal incorporation of nucleotides into DNA, a marker of immature cells of lymphoid and, to a lesser extent, myeloid lineages; early and common thymocytes are positive; haematogones may be positive. Expressed by the blast cells of most cases of B-ALL and T-ALL and the blast cells of about 15–20% of cases of AML; expression is weaker in AML; the neoplastic cells of acute promyelocytic leukaemia are negative; expressed by some non-haemopoietic tumours; apparent expression in germ cell tumours appears to be a cross-reaction. Very useful in confirming that leukaemic cells are immature; can be detected within the nucleus by immunohistochemistry and by flow cytometry after permeabilisation of the cells; useful for MRD monitoring in B-ALL, T-ALL and AML.

TIA-1

T cell-restricted intracellular antigen 1, a cytotoxic lymphocyte protein expressed in the cytoplasm of NK cells and cytotoxic T cells; often expressed by neutrophils. Used in immunohistochemistry but not often in flow cytometry as it is a cytoplasmic antigen.

TP53

The protein, p53, encoded by *TP53*, which is expressed in the nucleus of tumours of diverse origins.

von Willebrand factor

'Factor VIII-related antigen', expressed by megakaryocytes and endothelial cells. Sometimes used in immunohistochemistry to identify megakaryocytes and tumours of endothelial origin.

ZAP70

Expressed by thymocytes, T cells and NK cells. Expressed in a subset of cases of CLL, correlating with CD38 expression, absence of somatic *IGVH* mutation and a worse prognosis. Can be used for the categorisation of cases of CLL, with T cells and NK cells being excluded by gating.

Bibliography

Bain BJ (2017) *Leukaemia Diagnosis*, 5th edn, Wiley-Blackwell, Oxford.

Bain BJ, Clark DM and Wilkins BS (2019) *Bone Marrow Pathology*, 5th edn, Wiley-Blackwell, Oxford.

Gorczyca W (2017) *Flow Cytometry in Neoplastic Hematology: Morphologic-Immunophenotypic Correlation*, 3rd edn. CRC Press, Boca Raton.

Leach M, Drummond M and Doig A (2013), *Practical Flow Cytometry in Haematology Diagnosis*. Wiley-Blackwell, Oxford.

Leach M, Drummond M, Doig A, McKay P, Jackson R and Bain BJ (2015) *Practical Flow Cytometry in Haematology: 100 worked examples*. Wiley-Blackwell, Oxford.

Ortolani C (2011) *Flow Cytometry in Haematological Malignancies*, Wiley-Blackwell, Oxford.

Porwit A and Béné MC (2018) *Multiparameter Flow Cytometry in the Diagnosis of Hematologic Malignancies*, Cambridge University Press, Cambridge.

Sun T (2008) *Flow Cytometry and Immunohistochemistry for Hematologic Neoplasms*, Lippincott, Williams and Wilkins, Philadelphia.

Swerdlow SH, Campo E, Harris NL, Jaffe ES, Pileri S, Stein H and Thiele J (eds) (2017) *WHO Classification of Tumours of Haematopoietic and Lymphoid Tissues*, revised 4th edn. IARC Press, Lyon, pp. 37–38.

Torlakovic EE, Naresh KN and Brunning RD (2008) *Bone Marrow Immunohistochemistry*, ASCP, Chicago.

Websites

http://e-immunohistochemistry.info/web
https://en.wikipedia.org/wiki/ List_of_ human_clusters_of_differentiation
http://www.pathologyoutlines.com/cdmarkers.html
https://www.agilent.com/en/product/immunohistochemistry/antibodies-controls

Part 3

Immunophenotyping in the Diagnosis and Monitoring of Haematological Neoplasms and Related Conditions with Tables and Figures for Quick Reference

CONTENTS

Abbreviations

ALL, acute lymphoblastic leukaemia; AML, acute myeloid leukaemia; AMoL, acute monoblastic/monocytic leukaemia; APL, acute promyelocytic leukaemia; c, cytoplasmic; CD, cluster of differentiation; cIg, cytoplasmic immunoglobulin; CLL, chronic lymphocytic leukaemia; CMML, chronic myelomonocytic leukaemia; EBER, Epstein–Barr early RNA; EBNA, Epstein–Barr nuclear antigen; EBV, Epstein–Barr virus; EMA, epithelial membrane antigen; ETP-ALL, early T-cell precursor ALL; FSC, forward scatter; HHV, human herpesvirus; HLA, human leucocyte antigen; LMP, latent membrane protein; MDS, myelodysplastic syndrome; MDS/MPN, myelodysplastic/myeloproliferative syndrome; MPAL, mixed phenotype acute leukaemia; MPO, myeloperoxidase; MRD, minimal residual disease; NHL, non-Hodgkin lymphoma; NK, natural killer; PLL, prolymphocytic leukaemia; PNH, paroxysmal nocturnal haemoglobinuria; Sm, surface membrane; SmIg, surface membrane immunoglobulin; SSC, side scatter; TCR, T-cell receptor; TdT, terminal deoxynucleotidyl transferase.

Immunophenotyping for Haematologists: Principles and Practice, First Edition. Barbara J. Bain and Mike Leach.
© 2021 John Wiley & Sons Ltd. Published 2021 by John Wiley & Sons Ltd.

Normal Peripheral Blood and Bone Marrow Cells, Lineage and Stem Cell Markers

In Part 2, the expression of individual antibodies has been detailed. In Part 3, information has been assembled for quick reference in relation to specific diagnoses. Table 3.1 shows markers that are often studied and that are expressed by normal cells in the peripheral blood and bone marrow. When relevant, the strength of expression is shown as: – negative, ± weak, + moderate, ++ strong. Figures 3.1–3.5 show the alteration in expression of various markers with maturation within a lineage. The nature of the B-cell precursors known as haematogones and their distinction from neoplastic B lymphoblasts is discussed later.

Acute Myeloid Leukaemia

The major role of immunophenotyping in acute myeloid leukaemia (AML) is the recognition, as myeloid, of cases of acute leukaemia lacking cytological evidence of their lineage; this includes the recognition of monoblasts, megakaryoblasts and primitive erythroid cells as well as early myeloblasts that lack cytoplasmic granules or Auer rods. Other important roles are: (i) making a distinction from mixed phenotype acute leukaemia (MPAL); (ii) the identification of an immunophenotype that suggests a specific genetic subtype; and (iii) the identification of a leukaemia-associated immunophenotype that can be used for monitoring for minimal residual disease (MRD).

Table 3.2 shows antigens that are expressed in AML, including those that are associated with a specific genetic subtype.

Immunophenotype of Cells of Specific Myeloid Lineages

Myeloblasts typically express CD34, CD117, CD13, CD33, CD38, CD45 and CD133 and usually also myeloperoxidase (MPO) and human leucocyte antigen (HLA)-DR. Monoblasts express CD36, CD45, HLA-DR and CD64; they are MPO negative. Maturing cells of monocyte lineage express MPO, CD4, CD11a, CD11b, CD11c and CD14; there can also be expression of CD2, CD56, CD71 and CD123. Megakaryoblasts express CD41, CD42b and CD61; by immunohistochemistry, CD42b has been found to be most sensitive, followed by CD61, then von Willebrand antigen with immunohistochemistry for von Willebrand antigen yielding no further cases if CD42b and CD61 had been tested for [4] while CD36 is expressed but is not specific. Erythroblasts express glycophorin A (CD235a), which is lineage specific, together with CD36 and CD71, which are not lineage specific. E-cadherin can be detected by immunohistochemistry, permitting detection of earlier cells than those expressing glycophorin A and is erythroid-specific within haemopoietic lineages.

Correlation of Immunophenotype with Genotype

Specific immunophenotypic features can provide a clue to the underlying genetic abnormality [5]. This is particularly important in the identification of acute promyelocytic leukaemia, since rapid diagnosis and treatment can be crucial.

Acute promyelocytic leukaemia with t(15;17)(q24.1;q21.2); *PML-RARA* shows high side scatter (SCC), as a result of the granular cytoplasm, and expression of myeloid markers such as CD13 (heterogeneous), CD33 (strong), MPO and usually CD117; HLA-DR and CD34, which are usually expressed in AML, are generally negative although CD34 may be expressed in the microgranular variant; CD11b, CD11c, CD15, CD18 and CD16 are negative or weak; CD64 is often expressed; sometimes there is aberrant expression of CD2 and CD56 (about 10% of cases). CD9 is expressed in 95% of cases; CD9+CD11b–HLA-DR– has been found to have 85% sensitivity and 95% specificity for this diagnosis [6].

Table 3.1 Lineage and stem cell markers.

Cell type	Commonly used markers	Other markers	Markers that are generally negative
Neutrophil	CD11b++, CD11c+, CD13++, CD15++, CD16++, CD33±, CD38, CD45+, CD65+	CD10++, CD24++; CD64 is ± or – but upregulated during infection	CD34, CD117, HLA-DR
Eosinophil	CD11b++, CD11c+, CD13+, CD15+, CD33±, CD45++, high SSC	CD38+	CD34, CD117, HLA-DR, CD4, CD10, CD16
Basophil	CD9+, CD13+, CD33+, CD22±/+, CD123++, CD203c, CD45±*	CD25±/+, CD36+, CD38++	CD34, CD117, HLA-DR, CD64
Monocyte*	CD11b++, CD11c++, CD13++, CD14++†, CD15+‡, CD33++, CD45++, CD64++	HLA-DR variable, CD4±, CD36++, CD38++, CD300e on mature monocytes	CD34, CD117, CD16†
T lymphocyte	CD2+, SmCD3+, CD5+, CD7+, CD4+ or CD8+ (cytotoxic T cells are CD8+), CD43+, CD45++	CD56+ (minor population), CD57+ (minor population representing cytotoxic T cells), TCRαβ+ (majority of T cells), TCRγδ+ (minority of T cells)	CD25, HLA-DR (unless activated)
B lymphocyte	CD19+, CD20+, CD22+, CD79a+, CD79b+, surface membrane kappa or lambda+, HLA-DR+	Cytoplasmic immunoglobulin	CD5 (+ in mantle zone lymphocytes), CD23, CD38
NK cell§	CD2+, CD16§, CD56§, CD57+ or –§, CD45+	CD158a+¶, CD158b+¶, CD158+e¶	HLA-DR, CD3
Myeloid dendritic cell	CD45±, CD1c+, CD11c++, HLA-DR+, CD16 variable		
Plasmacytoid dendritic cell	CD45±, CD1c–, CD11c–, CD123++, HLA-DR+		
Mast cell	CD117++, CD9+, CD11c+, CD29+. CD33+, CD44+, CD45+, CD49d+. CD49e+, CD51+, CD54+, CD71+, CD38–, CD138–		
Plasma cell	CD19±, CD20–, CD22–, CD38++, CD138+/++, CD45 variable (–/±), cytoplasmic kappa or lambda+, SmIg–, CD56–, CD117–		CD56, CD117
Erythroblast	CD235a+/++, CD36+, CD71+, E-cadherin+		CD45
Haemopoietic stem cell	CD45±, CD34+, CD38+/–	CD49f+, CD90+	

Abbreviations: HLA, human leucocyte antigen; Sm, surface membrane; SSC, side scatter (of light); TCR, T-cell receptor
* There are conflicting data on the strength of expression.
† Classical monocytes, the major population in health, are CD14++, CD16–, non-classical are CD14+, CD16++, and there are intermediate forms.
‡ But weaker than on neutrophils.
§ NK cells are either (i) CD56++, CD16– /± or (ii) CD56±, CD16++ (more mature cells of this subset may also be CD57+).
¶ Heterogeneous expression on normal polyclonal NK cells.

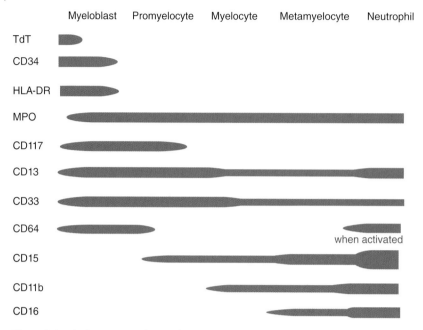

Figure 3.1 Antigen expression during maturation of the neutrophil lineage within the bone marrow. In addition, CD65 is expressed from the promyelocyte stage onwards and CD10 and CD24 on mature neutrophils. MPO, myeloperoxidase; TdT, terminal nucleotidyl transferase.

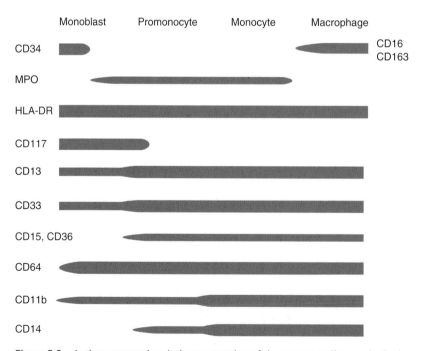

Figure 3.2 Antigen expression during maturation of the monocyte lineage in the bone marrow and, in tissues, to macrophages. In addition, CD4 is expressed at all stages of maturation.

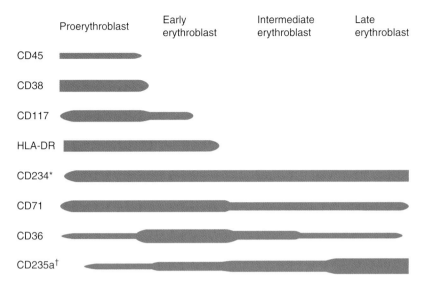

* E-cadherin
† Glycophorin A

Figure 3.3 Antigen expression during maturation of the erythroid lineage in the bone marrow. CD34 is not expressed by proerythroblasts.

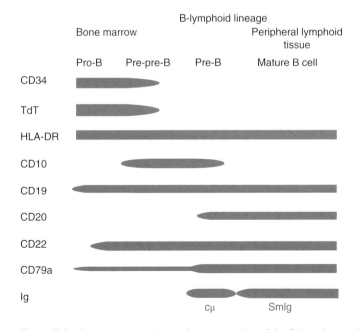

Figure 3.4 Antigen expression during maturation of the B-lymphocyte lineage in the bone marrow and in peripheral lymphoid tissues. For CD79a, it is a cytoplasmic epitope that is detected by flow cytometry. cμ, cytoplasmic μ chain; Ig, immunoglobulin; SmIg, surface membrane immunoglobulin.

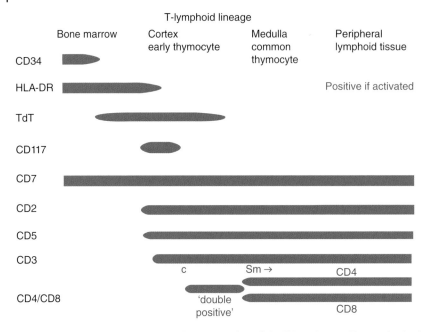

Figure 3.5 Antigen expression during maturation of the T-lymphocyte lineage in the bone marrow, thymus and peripheral lymphoid tissues. In addition, CD10 is expressed by the earliest recognised T-cell precursors. Early thymocytes are CD3 negative and it can thus be deduced that the bone marrow precursor of the T-lineage is also CD3 negative. A leukaemia derived from such a precursor would be classified as undifferentiated since expression of CD3 is necessary to define T lineage. c, cytoplasmic. (*Source:* from ref. [1])

CD56 is expressed in ≥20% of leukaemic pro-myelocytes in 10% of cases and is prognostically adverse, correlating with more induction deaths, a higher rate of relapse and lower overall survival [7].

AML with t(8;21)(q22;q22.1); *RUNX1-RUNX1T1* shows expression of CD34, HLA-DR and myeloid markers. Maturation can lead to expression of CD15 and CD65. Aberrant expression of CD19 (weaker than in B-lineage acute lymphoblastic leukaemia), CD79a, PAX5 and sometimes CD56 can be present, such expression being useful in the detection of MRD.

AML with inv(16)(p13.1q22) or t(16;16) (p13.1;q22); *CBFB-MYH11* usually shows expression of monocytic markers such as CD4, CD14, CD36 and CD38, sometimes markers of the neutrophil lineage such as CD15 and CD65, and often aberrant expression of CD2.

AML with t(9;11)(p21.3;q23.3); *KMT2A-MLLT3* usually shows expression of CD4, CD9, CD13 (weak), CD33, CD38, CD65, CD123, HLA-DR and NG2 (detected by the 7.1 antibody); CD15 and terminal deoxynucleotidyl transferase (TdT) are often positive; CD11b, CD11c, CD14, CD36 and CD64 may be expressed.

AML with t(6;9)(p23;q34.1); *DEK-NUP214* usually shows expression of CD9, CD13, CD15, CD33, CD34, CD38, CD117, CD123 and HLA-DR.

AML with inv(3)(q21.3q26.2) or t(3;3) (q21.3;q26.2); *GATA2, MECOM* can express CD7 and CD56 in addition to CD34, HLA-DR, CD13, CD33, CD65 and CD117. When there is megakaryocytic differentiation, there can be expression of CD41, CD42 and CD61. CD7 can be aberrantly expressed.

Table 3.2 Immunophenotyping of acute myeloid leukaemia and blastic plasmacytoid dendritic cell neoplasm.

Marker	Expression
CD34	Usually positive on blast cells except in AMoL, some cases of AML with *NPM1* mutation, some pure erythroid leukaemia and most acute megakaryoblastic leukaemias; usually negative in APL
HLA-DR	Usually positive except in APL, AML with *NPM1* mutation, some pure erythroid leukaemia and some acute megakaryoblastic leukaemia
CD45	Common leucocyte antigen; useful for gating on blast cells as expression is often weaker than on lymphocytes; often more strongly expressed by monoblasts than myeloblasts; megakaryoblasts are often negative; generally negative in pure erythroid leukaemia
Myeloperoxidase	Positive except in AML with minimal evidence of differentiation, acute megakaryoblastic leukaemia and pure erythroid leukaemia
CD117	Positive; may be negative in AMoL and weak in acute megakaryoblastic leukaemia
CD13	Positive
CD33	Positive; expression is relevant to monoclonal antibody treatment
CD11a	May be positive in AML, particularly with monocytic differentiation but not in APL; may be positive in acute megakaryoblastic leukaemia but not in cases with Down's syndrome or in transient abnormal myelopoiesis
CD11b, CD11c	Strongly expressed by normal monocytes; positive in AML when there is monocytic differentiation with maturing cells; can be expressed, more weakly, when there is granulocytic differentiation
CD14	Strongly expressed by normal monocytes; positive in AML when there is monocytic differentiation with maturing cells; variably positive on promonocytes but often negative on monoblasts
CD15	Positive when there is granulocytic or monocytic differentiation; more weakly expressed on neutrophils than monocytes
CD16	Positive on mature cells when there is granulocytic differentiation
CD64	Strongly expressed by normal monocytes; positive in AML when there is monocytic differentiation; often weakly positive in APL, both classical and variant, with heterogeneous distribution; may be weakly positive in acute megakaryoblastic leukaemia
CD65	Positive when there is granulocytic differentiation and sometimes when there is monocytic differentiation
CD36	Positive when there is monocytic differentiation and in pure erythroid leukaemia and acute megakaryoblastic leukaemia
CD38	Often positive; positive on leukaemic stem cells [2]; usually positive in acute megakaryoblastic leukaemia
CD2	Positive in a minority of cases of classical APL; usually positive in variant APL; may be positive in AML with inv(16)
CD4	Expressed on maturing monocytes; positive in AML with monocytic differentiation and in a minority of cases of classical APL and somewhat more often in variant APL; expressed in blastic plasmacytoid dendritic cell neoplasm
CD10	Expressed by neutrophils

(Continued)

Table 3.2 (Continued)

Marker	Expression
CD41, CD42, CD61	Positive in megakaryoblasts
CD235a	Glycophorin A, expressed in pure erythroid leukaemia
CD7	Aberrantly expressed in some cases; expressed in two-thirds of blastic plasmacytoid dendritic cell neoplasm
CD56	May be aberrantly expressed; often positive in AML with t(8;21) and when there is monocytic differentiation; expressed in a minority of cases of APL, both variant and classical; may be expressed by megakaryoblasts
CD19	Can be aberrantly expressed in AML with t(8;21)
CD79a	Can be aberrantly expressed in AML with t(8;21)
CD71	Sometimes positive, particularly in pure erythroid leukaemia, when expression is characteristically strong, and acute megakaryoblastic leukaemia, when expression is moderate
CD25	Expressed in a minority of cases of AML and is prognostically adverse
CD123	Positive on leukaemic stem cells [2], sometimes positive on myeloblasts and monoblasts; positive in blastic plasmacytoid dendritic cell neoplasm
CD133	Positive on leukaemic stem cells [2], on myeloblasts and in APL; monoblasts are usually negative
CD200	Expression is prognostically adverse, including in cytogenetically normal cases [3]
CD43	Often positive in pure erythroid leukaemia
Terminal deoxynucleotidyl transferase	Positive in a minority of cases
E-cadherin	Positive in pure erythroid leukaemia
PAX5	Pan-B marker; can be aberrantly expressed in AML with t(8;21)
Epithelial membrane antigen (CD227)	Often positive in pure erythroid leukaemia

Abbreviations: AML, acute myeloid leukaemia; AMoL, acute monoblastic leukaemia; APL, acute promyelocytic leukaemia.

Acute megakaryoblastic leukaemia with t(1;22)(p13.3;q13.1); *RBM15-MKL1* characteristically occurs in infants. Immunophenotyping is important is permitting its rapid diagnosis. There is expression of megakaryocytic markers such as CD41, CD42 and CD61 and, by immunohistochemistry, von Willebrand factor. CD13, CD33 and CD36 may be expressed while CD34 and HLA-DR are often negative.

AML with *NPM1* mutated can have an 'APL-like' immunophenotype, with CD34, HLA-DR or both being negative, CD33 being strong and CD13 often being weak; CD133 is also usually negative while CD110 and CD123 are often positive; some cases express monocytic markers – CD14, CD36 and CD64. CD19 can be aberrantly expressed. On immunohistochemistry, NPM1 is inappropriately expressed in the cytoplasm rather than the nucleus. A monoclonal antibody that recognises mutant NPM1 is available and can be used for monitoring MRD [8].

AML with biallelic *CEBPA* mutation usually shows expression of CD34, CD117, CD15, CD64, HLA-DR and strong MPO with asynchronous expression of CD15 and CD65 and aberrant expression of CD7 and CD56 being common [9, 10]. CD14 is generally not expressed. CD64 can be asynchronously expressed by neutrophils.

AML with mutated *RUNX1* usually shows expression of CD13, CD34, HLA-DR and CD13 and often expression of CD33 with variable expression of MPO and monocytic markers; expression of CD15, CD19 and CD56 is less common than in other categories of AML [11].

AML with myelodysplasia-related changes and **therapy-related AML** have variable immunophenotypic features.

AML, not otherwise specified has a variable immunophenotype, depending on differentiation. Pure erythroid leukaemia shows expression of CD36, CD71, CD117, CD235a and E-cadherin with HLA-DR, CD34 and CD45 usually being negative. Acute megakaryoblastic leukaemia shows expression of platelet glycoproteins and CD36 with CD34, CD45 and HLA-DR often being negative; CD7 can be aberrantly expressed. Acute basophilic leukaemia usually shows expression of CD9, CD11b, CD13, CD33, CD123 and CD203c but not CD117.

Transient abnormal myelopoiesis of Down's syndrome; *GATA1* mutated shows variable co-expression of stem cell and early myeloid markers (CD34 and CD117), myeloid markers (CD13 and CD33) and megakaryocyte markers (CD41, CD42 and CD61) with often aberrant expression of CD7 or CD56 [12]. CD13 and CD11b are often not expressed [13]. There is also usually expression of CD4 (weak), CD36, CD71, CD110 (the thrombopoietin receptor) and HLA-DR.

AML associated with Down's syndrome has a similar immunophenotype to that of transient abnormal myelopoiesis except that CD34 is negative in about half of cases and CD13 and CD11b are often expressed [13].

Acute Lymphoblastic Leukaemia, Mixed Phenotype Acute Leukaemia and Undifferentiated Acute Leukaemia

Immunophenotyping is crucial in confirmation of the diagnosis of acute lymphoblastic leukaemia (ALL), in distinguishing between B-lineage and T-lineage cases, and in making a distinction from MPAL. The distinction of early T-cell precursor ALL from other T-ALL is also important. Immunophenotyping is applicable to MRD monitoring.

Table 3.3 shows antigens that are expressed by normal T and B lymphocytes and those that can be applied to the diagnosis and further categorisation of ALL.

B-lineage Acute Lymphoblastic Leukaemia

Cases of B-ALL usually express CD19, CD79a (cytoplasmic epitope detected), often CD34 and often CD45 (can be weak or negative), TdT, HLA-DR and PAX5; they often express CD10 and CD22 (initially cytoplasmic) and sometimes CD20 or cytoplasmic μ chain. CD200 is expressed in about two-thirds of patients and CD56 in about 10%. Four stages of maturation are recognised, these showing some correlation with genetic subtypes. A mature B immunophenotype [17] is very rare (Table 3.4). Expression of myeloid antigens, such as CD13 and CD33, is common, and is applicable to MRD monitoring. On immunohistochemistry, PAX5 and CD79a are most often used for lineage assignment (but PAX5 can also be expressed in AML with t(8;21) and CD79a can be expressed in T-ALL). CD19 expression can be lost after CD19-targeted therapy.

B-ALL with high hyperdiploidy characteristically has the immunophenotype of common ALL. Approaching two-thirds of cases

Table 3.3 Immunophenotyping of normal mature T and B cells and in acute lymphoblastic leukaemia.

Marker	Normal expression and expression in ALL
SmCD3	Mature T cells and some T-ALL
cCD3	Mature and immature T cells and T-ALL
CD1a	Common thymocytes and about a third of cases of T-ALL
CD2	Mature T cells and most T-ALL
CD5	Mature T cells and most T-ALL
CD7	Normal mature T cells and T-ALL, aberrantly expressed in 15–20% of cases of AML
CD4 and CD8	Normal mature T cells express CD4 or CD8; T-ALL can be CD4−CD8− (about half of cases), CD4+CD8+ (about a third of cases) or, least often, CD4+ or CD8+
CD10	Germinal centre B cells, a proportion of cases of B-ALL ('common ALL'); more weakly expressed in about a third of cases of T-ALL
CD13	Not expressed by normal lymphocytes, can be aberrantly expressed in B-ALL and T-ALL
CD15	Not expressed by normal lymphocytes, can be aberrantly expressed in B-ALL, particularly with *KMT2A* rearrangement
CD19	Normal B cells and B-ALL
CD20	Normal B cells; positive in some B-ALL with a more mature immunophenotype
CD22	Normal B cells; positive in the cytoplasm in B-ALL and in cases with a more mature immunophenotype also on the Sm
CD24	B cells and their precursors; most B-ALL but not those with *KMT2A* rearrangement; can be expressed in AML with monocytic differentiation
CD33	Not expressed by normal lymphocytes, can be aberrantly expressed in B-ALL (particularly with *KMT2A* rearrangement) and T-ALL
CD34	Normal haemopoietic and lymphoid stem cells; usually positive in B-ALL (about 70% of cases) and AML, often positive in T-ALL
CD38	Haemopoietic stem cells, T-ALL including early precursor T-ALL [14], some B-ALL
CD45	Normal B and T cells and their precursors; often weak or even negative in B-ALL; generally more strongly expressed in T-ALL than in B-ALL but expression is weaker than that of mature T cells; weaker expression by lymphoblasts than by lymphocytes makes CD45 useful for gating on blast cells
CD56	Not expressed by normal B cells; expressed by NK cells and subsets of CD4-positive and CD8-positive T cells; expressed in a minority of cases of T-ALL
CD65	Can be aberrantly expressed in B-ALL, particularly with *KMT2A* rearrangement
CD71	Expressed by a minority of cases of B-ALL; more often expressed in T-ALL
CD79a	Expressed by normal and neoplastic B cells and their precursors; expressed in B-ALL; can be weakly expressed by T lymphoblasts [15,16]
CD117	Not expressed by normal lymphocytes; can be aberrantly expressed in T-ALL
CD123	Often positive in B-ALL; can be positive in T-ALL
CD200	Positive in B cells, a subset of T cells and in B-ALL
cµ	Positive in a subset of B-ALL ('pre-B ALL')
SmIg	Expressed by normal mature B cells; generally negative in B-ALL
TdT	Positive in B- and T-cell precursors; usually positive in B-ALL and T-ALL
HLA-DR	Positive in immature and mature B cells and B-ALL; not expressed by mature T cells; usually negative in T-ALL with the exception of early T-cell precursor ALL
CRLF2	Upregulated in some *BCR-ABL1*-like B-ALL
PAX5	Pan-B marker; can also be expressed in AML with t(8;21)

Abbreviations: ALL, acute lymphoblastic leukaemia; AML, acute myeloid leukaemia; c, cytoplasmic; Ig, immunoglobulin; Sm surface membrane; TdT, terminal deoxynucleotidyl transferase

Table 3.4 Maturation stages of B-lineage acute lymphoblastic leukaemia.

Maturation stage	Immunophenotypic characteristics	
Pro-B	CD19, cCD22, CD79a and HLA-DR almost always positive. TdT usually positive. CD45 may be weakly expressed or negative.	CD10−
Common ALL		CD10+
Pre-B		Cytoplasmic μ+, CD10 + or −
Mature B*		SmIg+

Abbreviations: c, cytoplasmic; SmIg, surface membrane immunoglobulin; TdT, terminal deoxynucleotidyl transferase.
* Very rare; cases of Burkitt lymphoma must be excluded.

express CD66c [18]. CD123 is often strongly expressed.

B-ALL with t(12;21)(p13.2;q22.1); *ETV6-RUNX1* characteristically has the immunophenotype of common ALL. CD27 is often expressed [19]. CD13 is often strongly expressed. There is rarely expression of CD9, CD20 or CD66c.

B-ALL with t(4;11)(q21.3;q23.3); *KMT2A-AFF1* often has a primitive, pro-B, immunophenotype with no expression of the common ALL antigen (CD10). There is characteristically expression of NG2, CD9 and often myeloid antigens, CD15, CD33, CD65 and CD123 [19]. Unlike most B-ALL, CD24 is not expressed.

B-ALL with t(9;22)(q34.1;q11.2); *BCR-ABL1* typically has a common ALL immunophenotype, expresses myeloid antigens, such as CD13 and CD33, and often expresses CD9, CD25 and CD123 [19]. Expression of CD66c is very common (about 80% of cases), expression of this antigen also being seen in about 60% of cases of high hyperdiploid ALL, in comparison with about 25% of other cases of B-ALL [18]. Expression of CD66c and aberrant myeloid antigens are applicable to MRD monitoring.

B-ALL with t(1;19)(q23;p13.3); *TCF3-PBX1* often has a pre-B immunophenotype (expression of cytoplasmic μ chain, and usually also CD10). Strong expression of CD9 is typical and CD34 is often negative.

BCR-ABL1-like ALL, which was initially defined by its gene expression profile, usually has a common ALL immunophenotype. Immunophenotyping can be useful in identifying those cases resulting from a translocation involving *CRLF2*, since there is increased expression of the protein.

Haematogones and Their Distinction from B Lymphoblasts

Haematogones are normal B-cell precursors. They are most prominent in the bone marrow of infants and children, on recovery from chemotherapy and following allogeneic bone marrow transplantation. As they have a precursor phenotype, it is very important to differentiate them from B lymphoblasts, particularly in patients following treatment for common ALL (CD19+, CD10+, CD20+/−). Haematogones are most prominent in healthy and regenerating marrows and tend to be markedly depleted in patients with primary bone marrow diseases such as the myelodysplastic syndromes, AML and aplastic anaemia. Morphologically, they have features intermediate between lymphoblasts and mature B cells, being of medium size with variably mature chromatin and sometimes nucleoli or nuclear clefts (Figure 3.6).

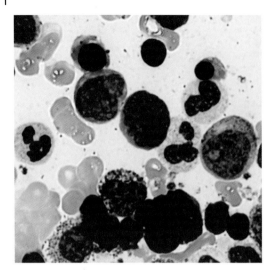
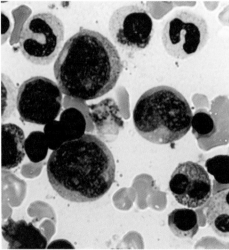

Figure 3.6 Bone marrow aspirate showing haematogones in a child during follow-up after an allogeneic transplant for B-ALL.

Regenerating marrows can show very prominent populations of haematogones (up to 20% of nucleated cells in some cases), so they can be easily confused with residual or relapsing disease.

There are three stages of maturation of haematogones, designated, depending on the degree of maturation within this precursor population, types I, II and III. Type I haematogones are the least mature often expressing CD34 and nuclear TdT together with CD19 and CD10. As they transition to type II cells, which normally make up the majority of the haematogone population, they lose CD34 and TdT, lose intensity of CD10 expression and gain CD20. It is important to note that type II haematogones often show a spectrum of CD20 expression. Type III cells start to lose CD10 and show more uniform CD20 expression. Mature B cells lose CD10 completely, show uniform CD20 positivity and gain surface immunoglobulin expression. By plotting marrow cells in a CD10 versus CD20 expression profile, it is usually possible to discriminate between common B-ALL blasts, the three types of haematogone and mature B cells (Figure 3.7a). Haematogone populations can also be identified using CD45 versus SSC characteristics as CD45 expression is also intermediate between that of normal B cells and B lymphoblasts/myeloblasts (Figure 3.7b).

By selectively gating on the haematogone zone and analysing the phenotype in relation to CD34, TdT, CD19, CD79a, CD10 and CD20, haematogones of various maturational stages can be accurately identified and separated from neoplastic precursor populations. Figure 3.8 shows the pattern of prominent haematogones in a marrow aspirate following allogeneic stem cell transplantation. The distribution of each subtype according to CD10 versus CD20 expression is illustrated in Figure 3.8b. Note the spectrum of CD20 expression in the type II cells and that in this case the small type III haematogone population is merging with mature B cells.

As haematogones always express CD10, it is particularly important to identify them as such in patients treated for common ALL. It is recommended that at diagnosis, the CD10 versus CD20 expression characteristics are recorded for future reference. Such a plot is illustrated in Figure 3.9 for a diagnostic specimen where the immunophenotype was CD19+, CD34+, CD79a+, TdT+, CD10++ and CD20−.

(a)

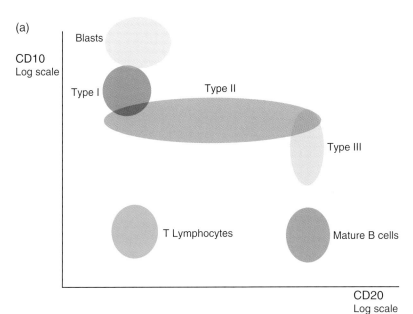

(b)

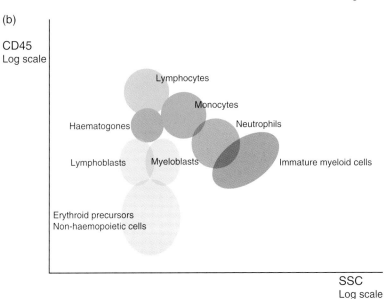

Figure 3.7 Flow cytometric immunophenotyping: (a) CD10 versus CD20 plot demonstrating the position of B lymphoblasts, haematogone subtypes and mature B cells; (b) utilisation of CD45 versus SSC to gate and help identify haematogones.

Typically, common ALL cells express strong CD10 and, regardless of the degree of CD20 expression, this helps to confirm clearance of such cells and separates them from haematogones in follow-up bone marrow aspirates. If patients are transferred between centres for allogeneic transplantation and this diagnostic data is not available, the assessment of post-transplant samples can prove to be substantially more difficult. Since pro-B-ALL does not express CD10, the discrimination of residual blasts from haematogones in this disease should

(a)

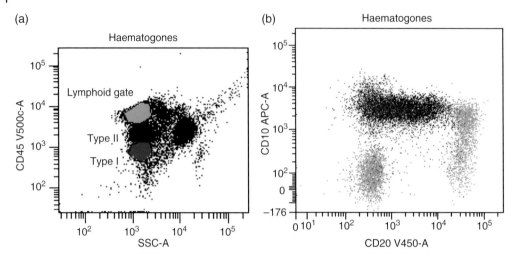

Figure 3.8 Flow cytometric immunophenotyping showing haematogones: (a) gating on haematogones type I and II according to CD45 expression; (b) haematogone subtype distribution in relation to CD10 and CD20 expression.

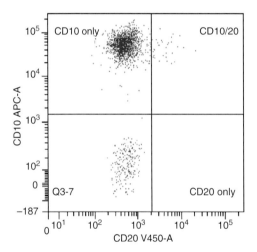

Figure 3.9 Flow cytometric immunophenotyping showing typical CD10 and CD20 expression at diagnosis in a patient with common ALL.

be straightforward. Pre-B-ALL often does not show CD34 and TdT expression so discrimination from type II haematogones is important. The assessment of any given patient relies on a multitude of factors including morphology, flow cytometry and cytogenetic and molecular MRD data. The key immunophenotypic elements used in the identification of haematogones and their discrimination from common B-ALL blasts are summarised in Table 3.5.

Finally, as noted above, it is important to appreciate that type II haematogones normally form the majority of the total haematogone population. In particular, if there appears to be an excess of type I haematogones, a careful scrutiny of the exact phenotype at diagnosis and comparison with all other response assessment data is absolutely essential.

T-lineage Acute Lymphoblastic Leukaemia

T-ALL usually shows expression of CD2, cytoplasmic (c) CD3, CD5, CD7, TdT and CD34, and sometimes of CD1a, CD10 (weak) and surface membrane (Sm) CD3; CD4−CD8− is most often observed followed by CD4+CD8+ and least often positivity for either CD4 or CD8 alone. TdT and CD99 are expressed. Four maturation stages are recognised (Table 3.6). In addition to weak CD10, markers that can be aberrantly expressed include CD79a, CD13 and CD33.

Among cases of T-ALL, early T-cell precursor ALL (ETP-ALL) must be distinguished due to its prognostic significance. It has been described by the WHO specialist group and others: there is expression of CD3 (cytoplasmic

Table 3.5 Typical immunophenotypic characteristics of common ALL cells compared with those of haematogones.

Antigen	Common-ALL lymphoblasts	Haematogones
CD10	Strong	Moderate/strong, type I
		Moderate, type II
		Weak, type III
CD20	Negative or variable	Negative type I
		Variable type II
		Positive type III
CD34	Often positive	Positive type I only
TdT	Often positive	Positive type I only
CD45	Weak or negative	Weak type I
		Intermediate type II
		Positive type III

Abbreviations: ALL, acute lymphoblastic leukaemia; TdT, terminal deoxynucleotidyl transferase

Table 3.6 Maturation stages of T-lineage acute lymphoblastic leukaemia.

Maturation stage	Immunophenotypic characteristics	
Pro-T*	CD7 is usually positive and is the earliest surface marker expressed; cCD3+, TdT usually positive (expression can be lost in later stages)	CD1a−, CD2−, CD4−, CD8−
Pre-T		CD1a−, CD2+, CD5+, CD4−, CD8−
Cortical T		CD4 and CD8+, CD1a+
Medullary T		CD4 or CD8+, CD1a−

Abbreviations: c, cytoplasmic; TdT, terminal deoxynucleotidyl transferase
* Cases of early T-cell precursor ALL must be distinguished (see text).

and rarely membrane) and usually of CD2 and CD7; CD1a, CD4 and CD8 are not usually expressed, and there is expression of one or more of CD34, CD117, HLA-DR, CD13, CD33, CD11b, CD15 and CD65; CD5 is usually weak or negative. The WHO definition [20] requires negativity for CD1a and CD8 and expression of one or more of CD34, CD117, CD11b, CD13, CD33, CD65 and HLA-DR. CD2 and TdT are less likely to be expressed than in other T-ALL and CD10 is much less likely to be expressed [21]. CD45 is usually negative or weak. A scoring system based on 11 immunophenotypic markers (Table 3.7) has been found to give reliable identification of ETP-ALL with all cases scoring at least 8 and other T-ALL having a score of less than 7 [21].

In the case of a mediastinal tumour it may be necessary to distinguish between T-ALL and a thymoma, an epithelial tumour which, particularly in children, can be rich in immature reactive lymphoid cells, which can express TdT. Misdiagnosis is possible [22]. The presence of CD4-positive, CD8-positive and double positive lymphoid cell populations is seen in thymoma but not T-ALL, which generally has a single homogeneous population (rarely T-ALL has a subset of cells with a somewhat

Table 3.7 A scoring system for the identification of early T-cell precursor acute lymphoblastic leukaemia (*Source:* from ref. [21], with permission of the British Journal of Haematology).

Marker	Expressed*	Not expressed
CD1a	−2	2
SmCD3	−2	
CD5	−2	2
CD8		2
CD10		1
CD13	1	
CD33	1	
CD34	1	
CD117	1	
TdT		1
MPO	−1	

Abbreviations: MPO, myeloperoxidase; Sm, surface membrane; TdT, terminal deoxynucleotidyl transferase
* Cut-off of 20% for expression except for CD5 for which the cut-off is 75%.

different immunophenotype from the dominant population). Weak or negative CD45 with an abnormal phenotype, such as CD4+ CD8+ CD3− CD10+ with aberrant myeloid markers identifies T-ALL. Immunohistochemical demonstration of cytokeratin and E-cadherin expression is useful to demonstrate sparse thymic epithelial cells [22].

Acute Mixed Phenotype Leukaemia and Acute Undifferentiated Leukaemia

Immunophenotyping is essential for the diagnosis of MPAL. Table 3.8 shows markers that are required for this diagnosis, as defined in the 2016 WHO classification [23]. It should be noted that although expression of CD13 or CD33 is not sufficient for the identification of myeloid differentiation in suspected MPAL, such expression can be considered sufficient to define a very early myeloid leukaemia when no specific lymphoid markers are expressed.

Acute undifferentiated leukaemia is diagnosed when there is no expression of lineage-specific markers; markers that may be

expressed are CD7, CD34, CD38, CD45, HLA-DR and TdT.

Myelodysplastic Syndromes and Myelodysplastic/ Myeloproliferative Neoplasms

Aberrant, asynchronous and under- or over-expression of antigens and abnormal light scatter have been used as diagnostic aids in the myelodysplastic syndromes (MDS) and myelodysplastic/myeloproliferative neoplasms (MDS/MPN), including chronic myelomonocytic leukaemia (CMML) (Table 3.9). Hypogranularity of neutrophils leads to reduced SSC (Figure 3.10). Monocytes can show increased SSC. Antigens that can be under-expressed by neutrophils include CD10, CD11b, CD13 and CD16. CD117 can be asynchronously expressed on mature neutrophils. CD56 can be aberrantly expressed on neutrophils and monocytes. CD10, CD16 and CD23 can be aberrantly expressed on monocytes. The European LeukemiaNet has recommended a scoring system for the identification of

Table 3.8 Markers that are required for the definition of mixed phenotype acute leukaemia.*

Marker†	Significance	Lineage
MPO	Defines myeloid, particularly granulocytic, lineage‡	Myeloid
	OR	
CD11c, CD14, CD64, lysozyme	Expression of at least two of these defines monocytic lineage§	
cCD3 (or SmCD3)	Defines T lineage	T-cell
CD19	If strong, together with strong expression of at least one of CD10, cCD22, CD79a.	B-cell
	If weak, together with strong expression of at least two of CD10, cCD22, CD79a.	
CD10	See above	
cCD22	See above	
CD79a	See above	

Abbreviations: c, cytoplasmic; MPO, myeloperoxidase; Sm, surface membrane
* Cases with t(8;21), which would otherwise fit these criteria, are excluded.
† These markers can be combined with CD45 (together with SSC) for gating, and with markers of immaturity (CD34, terminal deoxynucleotidyl transferase).
‡ Cytochemical demonstration of myeloperoxidase is an alternative.
§ Cytochemical demonstration of non-specific esterase is an alternative.

low-grade MDS, based on the work of Ogata and colleagues [24], which shows 69% sensitivity and 92% specificity [25]. The four variables incorporated are: an increased CD34-positive myeloblast-related cluster; reduced B-cell progenitors; increased or reduced CD45 expression on myeloblasts; and reduced granulocyte SSC. In a further evaluation, sensitivity was 75.6% and specificity, 91.2% [26].

CD14 and CD16 have been found useful in the diagnosis of CMML: about 85% of monocytes in healthy subjects are 'classical monocytes' (CD14+CD16−), the others being intermediate (CD14+CD16+) or non-classical (CD14^{weak}CD16+); CMML is characterised by more than 94% classical monocytes [27, 28]. A decrease in the percentage of non-classical monocytes has a similar sensitivity and specificity [29]. Aberrantly expressed antigens in CMML include CD56 (80% of cases), CD2 (10–40%) and CD10 and CD23 (both about a quarter of cases), but aberrant antigen expression can also occur in reactive monocytosis [29]. Reduced

expression of CD11c has been found to have a high specificity for CMML with a sensitivity of 70% [29]. Reduced expression of other antigens, including HLA-DR, can also occur but is not specific for neoplasia [29]. Immunohistochemistry for CD14, CD68R and CD163 can demonstrate monocytic differentiation and may also show a population of plasmacytoid dendritic cells.

Atypical chronic myeloid leukaemia, like CMML, shows an increased percentage of classical monocytes and a decreased percentage of non-classical ones [29]. Monocytic differentiation can be demonstrated, as above, by immunohistochemistry but immunophenotyping is not important in diagnosis.

The detection of a small paroxysmal nocturnal haemoglobinuria (PNH) clone, for example with lack of expression of CD55, CD59 or reduced FLAER binding (see below), can also strengthen the diagnosis of MDS. Haematogones are decreased in MDS. There is upregulation of CD200, expression being prognostically adverse [30].

Table 3.9 Markers that have been applied in the diagnosis of myelodysplastic syndromes and myelodysplastic/myeloproliferative neoplasms.

Marker	Application
CD2	Aberrant expression
CD5	Aberrant expression
CD7	Aberrant expression
CD10	Under-expression by neutrophils in MDS
CD11b, CD11c	Under-expression by neutrophils or monocytes; over-expression by neutrophils; expression by immature myeloid cells including blast cells in MDS
CD13	Under-expression by monocytes in CMML and MDS; under- or over-expression in MDS
CD14	Diagnosis of CMML (reduced expression; increased 'classical' monocytes)
CD15	Under-expression by monocytes in CMML; expression by immature myeloid cells including blast cells in MDS
CD16	Diagnosis of CMML (increased 'classical' monocytes); under-expression by neutrophils in MDS
CD19	Aberrant expression
CD33	Under-expression
CD34	Increased blast cells; asynchronous expression by maturing cells of neutrophil or monocyte lineage
CD36	Under-expression by erythroblasts and by monocytes in CMML
CD45	Reduced expression by blast cells or neutrophils
CD56	Aberrant expression including expression on blast cells and strong expression by monocytes in CMML
CD64	Under-expression by monocytes in CMML; expression by neutrophils in MDS
CD65	Aberrant expression on blast cells
CD71	Under-expression by erythroblasts
CD117	Expression on maturing cells
HLA-DR	Under-expression by monocytes in CMML; aberrant expression by myelocytes, metamyelocytes and neutrophils in MDS
SSC	Reduced for neutrophils, myelocytes, promyelocyte

Abbreviations: CMML, chronic myelomonocytic leukaemia; HLA, human leucocyte antigen; MDS, myelodysplastic syndrome; SSC, sideways scatter.

It should be noted that changes similar to those occurring in MDS and MDS/MPN can occur in reactive conditions such as infection, bone marrow regeneration and following the use of growth factors.

Myeloproliferative Neoplasms

Neoplastic cells of myeloproliferative neoplasms can show reduced SSC by neutrophils, downregulation of antigens (e.g. CD10, CD11b, CD15 or CD16 on neutrophils) and aberrant expression (e.g. of CD56 on neutrophils). However, other diagnostic modalities are of considerably more importance. The main role of immunophenotyping is in the identification of the lineage in blast transformation.

Systemic Mastocytosis

Neoplastic mast cells express CD117 and mast cell tryptase (strongly) in addition to CD43, CD45 and CD68; they differ from normal mast cells in expressing CD2 and CD25 and, when the disease

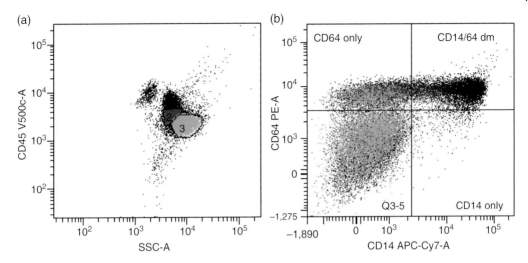

Figure 3.10 Flow cytometric immunophenotyping showing reduced granulocyte side scatter (SSC) in a patient with MDS. The gate on population 1 (blue) captures mature monocytes. Population 3 (green) represents the more granular neutrophils with increased SSC. The hypogranular neutrophils, population 2, (red) show reduced SSC and are merging with the monocyte population. They also show aberrant expression of CD64.

is aggressive, may express CD30. CD203c is expressed. CD123 has been reported to be aberrantly expressed in a quarter [31] and two-thirds [32] of cases. Flow cytometry has been found to be more sensitive than immunohistochemistry in the detection of CD2 and CD25 positivity [33], but it should be noted that an aspirate may not contain appreciable numbers of mast cells despite their being detected in trephine biopsy specimens. The mast cells in myeloproliferative neoplasms associated with *PDGFRA* and *PDGFRB* fusion genes can also express CD25 but less often CD2. In mast cell leukaemia there may be expression of CD34 [34].

Flow cytometric evidence of myelodysplasia is an independent adverse risk factor in systemic mastocytosis [35].

Blastic Plasmacytoid Dendritic Cell Neoplasm

The most characteristic markers are CD4, CD56, CD123 (stronger than in AML or ALL), CD303 (blood-derived dendritic cell antigen 2) and CD304 (blood-derived dendritic cell antigen 4). There is usually also expression of CD36, CD38, CD43, CD45 (weak), CD45RA, CD68, CD71, HLA-DR (strong), TCL1A and TCF4 and often expression of CD7 and CD33. There is sometimes expression of CD2, CD5, CD34, CD79a, CD117, S100 and TdT. Expression of TdT has been found to be prognostically favourable [36]. In one series CD3 was expressed in 10 of 55 patients studied [36]. Expression of granzyme B may be detected by flow cytometry but, on immunohistochemistry, is either negative or shows only dot positivity rather than diffuse cytoplasmic positivity [37].

Langerhans Cell Histiocytosis and Erdheim–Chester Disease

The diagnosis of Langerhans cell histiocytosis is generally made histologically. There is usually expression of CD1a, CD4, CD14, CD40, CD45, CD52, CD64, CD68, CD207 (langerin), CD274 (PD-L1), HLA-DR, S100 and vimentin [38]. The closely related Erdheim–Chester disease shows expression of CD14, CD68 and CD163 and, when the relevant mutation is present, expression of BRAF V600E occurs. CD1a and CD207 are not expressed; S100 is expressed in 10–30% of cases [37].

Histiocytic Sarcoma

There is expression of CD11c, CD14, CD68, CD163, lysozyme, often CD274 and, in about half of cases, S100 [37].

Mature B-lineage Neoplasms

Immunophenotyping is important in confirming a diagnosis of a B-cell neoplasm and in distinguishing neoplasms of mature B cells from reactive conditions and from ALL. Immunophenotyping often points to a specific diagnosis, can sometimes give prognostic information, and is applicable to MRD monitoring. In the case of chronic lymphocytic leukaemia (CLL) and hairy cell leukaemia, the characteristic immunophenotypes have a high degree of specificity for the diagnosis.

Table 3.10 shows a panel of antibodies that can be used to characterise mature B-lineage neoplasms. Identification of clonality requires the use of anti-κ and anti-λ antibodies, which

Table 3.10 Characteristic immunophenotype of chronic B-cell leukaemias and B-cell lymphomas that can involve the peripheral blood [39–41].

Marker	CLL	PLL	HCL	Follicular lymphoma*	Mantle cell lymphoma†	SMZL/ SLVL	Plasma cell leukaemia
SmIg	Weak	Strong	Strong or moderate	Strong	Moderate	Strong	Negative
cIg	−	−/+	−/+	−	−	−/+	++
CD5	++	−/+	−	−	++	−	−
CD19, CD20, CD24, CD79a	++‡	++	++§	++	++	++	−
CD79b	−	++	−/+	++	++	++	−
CD23	++	−	−	−/+	−/+	−/+	−
FMC7, CD22	−/+	++	++	++	+	++	−
CD10	−	−/+	−	+	−/+	−	−/+
CD11c	−/+	++	++	−	−/+	+	?
CD25	−/+	−	++	−	−	−/+	−
CD38	−/+	−	−/+	−/+	−	−/+	++
CD43	+	−/+	−	−	+	−/+	+
CD200	++	−	++	−	−	−/+	−/+
HLA-DR	++	++	++	++	++	++	−
IRF4/MUM1	+	?	−	−/+	−/+	−/+	++

The frequency with which a marker is positive in >30% of cells in a particular leukaemia is indicated as follows: ++, 80–100%; +, 40–80%; −/+, 10–40%; −, 0–9%.
CLL, chronic lymphocytic leukaemia; cIg, cytoplasmic immunoglobulin; HCL, hairy cell leukaemia; HLA, human leucocyte antigen; PLL, prolymphocytic leukaemia; SLVL, splenic lymphoma with villous lymphocytes; SmIg, surface membrane immunoglobulin; SMZL, splenic marginal zone lymphoma.
* Follicular lymphoma cells express BCL2 whereas germinal centre cells of reactive follicular hyperplasia are negative; BCL2 and CD10 expression is less frequent in higher-grade follicular lymphoma [41].
† The minority of cases of mantle cell lymphoma that are leukaemic, non-nodal with mutated *IGVH* genes are less likely to express CD5, and are much more often CD200 positive.
‡ CLL cells express CD20 fairly weakly.
§ HCL cells are negative with at least some monoclonal antibodies of the CD24 cluster.
Source: from refs. [39–41].

will also permit assessment of the strength of expression of surface membrane immunoglobulin (SmIg). For an economical use of reagent antibodies, it can be useful to use an initial panel to establish lineage and clonality, and to distinguish CLL from other neoplasms of mature B cells and from T-lineage neoplasms, followed by more specialised panels to further elucidate the diagnosis.

Chronic Lymphocytic Leukaemia

In CLL, the neoplastic cells express B-lineage markers such as CD19, CD20, CD22, CD79a and SmIg (Table 3.10). Expression of CD20, CD22 and SmIg tends to be weak. In addition, CLL cells express CD5, CD23, CD43 and CD200; there is weak expression of CD11c and negative or weak expression of CD79b and FMC7. Scoring systems including four (CD5, CD23, CD200 and SmIg) [42] or five (CD5, CD23, CD22/CD79b, FMC7 and SmIg [43] or CD5, CD23, CD79b, FMC7 and CD200 [44]) markers are effective at distinguishing CLL from other neoplasms of mature B cells. ROR1 is expressed. CD274 (PD-1) is not expressed [45]. CD54 may be expressed and is prognostically adverse [46, 47]. Immunohistochemistry shows expression of LEF1, which is not expressed by normal B cells or in most other mature B-cell neoplasms. Cyclin D1 and SOX11 are not expressed.

A collaboration of two expert groups (ERIC and ESCCA) led to the recommendation of an essential panel comprising CD19, CD5, CD20, CD23, kappa and lambda, and a recommended panel that is potentially useful for differential diagnosis, comprising CD43, CD79b, CD81, CD200, CD10 and ROR1 [48].

Immunophenotyping is not only distinctive, thus being crucial in diagnosis, but also gives prognostic information. Expression of CD38, ZAP70 and CD49b are prognostically adverse, as is weak rather than strong expression of CD5 [49]. MUM1/IRF4 expression, seen in about half of patients, is prognostically adverse [50].

Mantle Cell Lymphoma

Mantle cell lymphoma, like other B-cell non-Hodgkin lymphoma (NHL), shows expression of pan-B markers (CD19, CD20, CD22 and CD79a), typically also CD5 [51] and CD43 and sometimes CD10. CD5 expression is absent in a small subset of cases, particularly in the blastoid variant [52]. Mantle cell lymphoma differs from CLL in expressing FMC7 and CD79b, in having moderate rather than weak expression of SmIg and in usually being negative for CD23 and CD200. CD200 expression is more likely in the leukaemic, non-nodal variant. Nuclear cyclin D1 expression, resulting from dysregulation of *CCND1* by t(11;14) or a related translocation, can be detected by flow cytometry of permeabilised cells or by immunohistochemistry in the majority of cases; when not detected, nuclear expression of SOX11 is useful in confirming the diagnosis. Immunohistochemistry or flow cytometry for ROR1 expression has been suggested for the differential diagnosis of CD5-positive B-cell neoplasms; however, as is strongly expressed in mantle cell lymphoma as well as in CLL, it does not appear to be very useful [53]. BCL2 is usually expressed but not BCL6. IRF4/MUM1 may be expressed [54]. CD274 (PD-1) is not expressed [45]. LEF1 is usually negative.

Follicular Lymphoma

Follicular lymphoma shows expression of pan-B markers including CD19, CD20, CD22, CD79a, CD79b and FMC7. The only distinctive marker is CD10, which is reliably detected in lymph node biopsies but is also often expressed by lymphoma cells in the peripheral blood or bone marrow. CD43, CD200 [39] and ROR1 [53] are not expressed. In histological sections, BCL2 expression is also useful since reactive lymphoid follicles are negative; it is often negative in grade III disease. BCL6 expression is usual and provides further evidence of germinal centre origin. Expression of MUM1/IRF4 is mainly seen in grade 3 follicular lymphoma. CD274 (PD-1) is not expressed [44].

In the small minority of patients (2–3%) with EBV-positive follicular lymphoma, immunohistochemistry demonstrates Epstein–Barr virus (EBV) latent membrane protein 1 (LMP1) but not EBV Nuclear Antigen 2 (EBNA2) [55].

Marginal Zone Lymphomas

Splenic, nodal and extranodal marginal zone lymphomas have no distinctive immunophenotypic features. Expression of CD200 is weaker than that of normal B cells [39] but in about a third of patients with nodal or extranodal marginal zone lymphoma, there is moderate to strong expression overlapping with that of CLL. CD274 (PD-1) is not expressed [45]. In one study IRF4/MUM1 was found to be expressed in 38% of extranodal marginal zone lymphomas [56]. In a study of a small number of patients, ROR1 expression was observed in circulating lymphoma cells but not in bone marrow cells, expression being weaker than in CLL and mantle cell lymphoma [53].

In trephine biopsy sections, immunohistochemistry for B-lineage antigens can highlight the intrasinusoidal infiltration that is characteristically part of the pattern of infiltration in splenic marginal zone lymphoma and can be seen, although less often, in nodal marginal zone lymphoma.

Lymphoplasmacytic Lymphoma/ Waldenström Macroglobulinaemia

There are usually monotypic lymphocytes and plasma cells but proportions vary between patients. Lymphocytes show expression of B-lineage markers (CD19, CD20, CD22, CD79a and CD79b), but CD22 expression may be weak [57]. There is not usually expression of CD5 (reports vary but a quarter of cases showed mainly partial positivity in one series [58]), CD10, CD23 (reports vary but a half of patients were positive in the same series [58]), CD43, CD103 or BCL6. FMC7 is often negative while CD11c, CD25 and CD38 are often positive. CD27 and CD52 are often expressed [57].

CD200 is sometimes expressed [39]. CD13 expression is more common than in other B-cell neoplasms, being expressed by more than 20% of cells in two-thirds of patients [59]. Immunohistochemistry shows cytoplasmic rather than nuclear staining for CXCR4 in approaching 40% of cases; this correlates with the prognostically adverse *CXCR4* mutation found in 30% of cases, although some non-mutated cases also show cytoplasmic staining [60]. Cells showing plasma cell differentiation express CD38, CD79a, CD138, MUM1/IRF4, PAX5 and cytoplasmic immunoglobulin (cIg) but lack the CD19 negativity and aberrant CD56 expression of myeloma and often express CD45 [57, 58]. The latter features are important in differentiating between lymphoplasmacytic lymphoma and rare cases of IgM myeloma.

Prolymphocytic Leukaemia

There is usually strong expression of SmIg and pan-B markers, CD19, CD20, CD22, CD79a and CD79b. FMC7 and CD11c are usually expressed while CD5, CD10, CD23, CD25 and CD200 are usually negative. If CD5 is expressed, it is important to exclude a diagnosis of mantle cell lymphoma, in which the cytological features of lymphoma cells sometimes resemble those of prolymphocytes. Around half of cases express CD38. As there is no specific immunophenotype, it is important that the morphological features of this condition are recognised at diagnosis and correlated with the clinical presentation.

Hairy Cell Leukaemia

Hairy cell leukaemia is readily diagnosed from the cytological and immunophenotypic features. CD19, CD20, CD22, CD200 and SmIg are usually strongly expressed, CD200 even more strongly than in CLL and B-ALL [39]. The most distinctive immunophenotypic features are expression of CD11c, CD25, CD103 and CD123; CD7, CD305 and FMC7 are also positive. CD10 is expressed in a minority of patients [61]. On immunohistochemical staining, tartrate-resistant acid phosphatase, annexin A1, DBA-44, cyclin D1 and, more specifically, BRAF V600E are also positive.

Immunophenotyping is relevant to treatment as well as diagnosis since BRAF inhibitors and a CD22-directed immunotoxin are applicable.

It is important to note that hairy cells often have forward scatter (FSC)/SSC characteristics similar to those of normal monocytes (Figure 3.11) and automated analysers may erroneously indicate a normal (or raised) monocyte count when in fact there is an actual monocytopenia, typical of classical hairy cell leukaemia. Clinicians may therefore fail to consider this diagnosis when considering the differential diagnosis in a patient presenting with cytopenias. As always, a careful review of the blood film is important.

Hairy Cell Leukaemia Variant

There is expression of pan-B markers. FMC7 is usually positive and CD5 and CD23 are negative [62]. CD79b is positive in about a third of cases [62]. Immunophenotypic features that help to distinguish hairy cell leukaemia vari-

ant from hairy cell leukaemia are negativity for CD25 and weak or absent expression of CD123, while CD11c and CD103 are likely to be positive. CD200 is usually negative [39, 62]. On immunohistochemistry, DBA-44 and PAX5 are positive; annexin A1, cyclin D1 and BRAF V600E are negative.

Splenic Diffuse Red Pulp Small B-cell Lymphoma

This lymphoma shows expression of CD19, CD20 and other pan-B markers, CD180 (diagnostically useful as expression is stronger than in other B-cell neoplasms) and FMC7, with usually absent expression of CD5, CD10, CD23, CD25 (3%), CD43, CD103 and CD123 [63]. CD11c may or may not be expressed. On immunohistochemistry, there is expression of DBA.44 but not annexin A1 or IRF4/MUM1. Immunohistochemistry permits appreciation of intrasinusoidal infiltration on bone marrow biopsy [63].

Burkitt Lymphoma

Burkitt lymphoma is readily diagnosed from the cytological or histological features, supplemented by the immunophenotype. There is usually a mature B-cell immunophenotype with expression of pan-B markers and strong SmIg, together with CD10, CD38, CD43 and CD71. CD200 is not expressed [39]. On immunohistochemical staining, there is also expression of PAX5, MYC and BCL6 while BCL2 is negative. MUM1/IRF4 is more often negative. CD274 (PD-1) is not expressed [45]. The expression of CD10 and BCL6 reflects the germinal centre origin of this lymphoma. CD21 expression correlates with EBV positivity. Rarely there is a precursor-B immunophenotype with expression of TdT and sometimes CD34, lack of expression of SmIg and sometimes lack of expression of CD20 [64]. The expression of Ki-67, a proliferation marker, is diagnostically very important as the proliferation fraction approaches 100%.

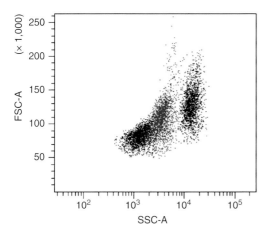

Figure 3.11 Forward scatter (FSC) versus side scatter (SSC) plot from a case of hairy cell leukaemia. The hairy cells (red) are distributed over the monocyte window and may be counted as such by automated analysers.

Diffuse Large B-cell Lymphoma

Diffuse large B-cell lymphoma expresses pan-B markers CD20, CD22, CD79, SmIg, PAX5 and also OCT2 and BOB1. CD30 is expressed in a minority of cases, particularly in EBV-positive cases. Genetic analysis has divided cases into prognostically significant groups, germinal centre B-cell-like (GCB) and activated B-cell-like (ABC), with some cases being unclassified. Several immunohisto-chemistry-based algorithms have been devised to seek to recognise these categories. In one, the expression of CD10 leads to a categorisation as GCB-like with cases expressing MUM1/IRF4 being non-GCB-type [65]. Others have used CD10, FOXP1 and BCL6 as indicators of a GCB-like lymphoma [66]. CD274 (PD-L1) may be expressed in the ABC-like subset [45] and MUM1/IRF4 expression is also associated with this category. The CD79b-directed antibody–drug conjugate, polatuzumab vedotin, has therapeutic potential.

Primary Mediastinal Large B-cell Lymphoma

This lymphoma shows expression of B-lineage markers and cytoplasmic but not SmIg; there is expression of CD19 and CD20 (strong) and usually expression of CD22, CD23 (2/3 of cases), CD79a, CD274 (PD-L1), BCL2, BCL6, IRF4/MUM1, PAX5, BOB1, OCT2 and weak or variable CD30 with CD10 and CD11c being less often expressed; CD15 is negative or weakly or focally positive. Low expression of CD274 (PD-L1) and high expression of IRF4/MUM1 have been found to be prognostically adverse [67]. The PD-1 inhibitor, pembrolizumab, has therapeutic potential.

Primary Effusion Lymphoma

Immunophenotyping of cells in serous fluid is useful in the diagnosis of this lymphoma; there is expression of CD38, CD43, CD45, CD54, CD71, CD138, IRF4/MUM1, HLA-DR, epithelial membrane antigen (EMA, CD227), human herpesvirus 8 (HHV8)-associated latent nuclear antigen 1 (LANA1), the antigen detected by VS38c, and often CD30 (~ 70%) [68]. There is no expression of CD19, CD20, CD79a, PAX5, cIg or SmIg. There can be aberrant expression of CD2, CD3, CD4 or CD5 [69]. There is co-infection with EBV in 80% of cases but EBV LMP1 is not expressed; EBV early RNA (EBER) may be detected.

HHV8-negative primary effusion lymphoma appears to be a distinct entity, which is indolent in its behaviour. There is a mature B-cell immunophenotype [70].

Intravascular Large B-cell Lymphoma

This lymphoma not infrequently involves the bone marrow, 60% of 43 patients in one study. In the same study, antigen expression was CD5 50%, CD10 17%, MUM1/IRF4 95%, BCL6 56% and BCL2 80% [71].

High-Grade B-cell Lymphoma with Rearrangement of *MYC* and *BCL2, BCL6* or both

There is expression of CD19, CD20, CD79a, PAX5 and usually BCL2 (particularly in cases with *BCL2* rearrangement) [72]. CD10 is usually positive. SmIg is sometimes not expressed. There is variable expression of CD10 and IRF4/MUM1 (respectively less frequent and more frequent in *BCL6* rearranged cases) [72]. Ki-67 expression can be high.

Plasmablastic Lymphoma

There is expression of CD38, CD138, CD319, MUM1/IRF4, the antigen detected by the VS38c antibody [73, 74] and often CD30 and EMA. CD79a may be expressed. CD56 and CD10 are expressed in a minority of cases. CD30 has been reported to be frequently [73] or infrequently [74] expressed. CD20, CD45 and PAX5 are generally negative. Some cases express CD10, CD43, CD56 or CD79a. Although cases are often EBV positive, EBV LMP1 is usually negative [73]. Ki-67 expression is high.

Persistent Polyclonal B-cell Lymphocytosis

This condition, seen particularly in female cigarette smokers, must be distinguished from B-cell neoplasms. There is expression of surface membrane IgM and IgD without light chain restriction. Typically there is also expression of CD19, CD20, CD22, CD79a and CD79b but not CD5 or CD10.

Plasma Cell Neoplasms

Multiple Myeloma (Plasma Cell Myeloma)

Immunophenotyping is applicable when there is difficulty making a diagnosis of multiple myeloma and for MRD monitoring. Table 3.11 [75–77] compares the usual immunophenotype of myeloma cells with that of normal plasma cells. Myeloma cells sometimes express EMA (CD227) or cyclin D1, the latter reflecting the presence of t(11;14) with dysregulation of *CCND1*. These cases are often CD20 positive. Exceptionally rarely, myeloma cells express both κ and λ light

Table 3.11 A comparison of the typical immunophenotype of normal plasma cells and myeloma cells.

	Normal plasma cells*	Myeloma cells*
CD38	+ (strong)	+ (weak in 80% of cases)
CD138	+	+ (tends to be stronger than in normal plasma cells)
CD319	+	+
CD19	+	96–97% −
CD20	−	15–20% +
CD45	Weak	− or weak (− in 89–96%)
CD56	−	76–96% +
CD79a	+	Weak or negative in about half of cases
CD30	+	−
CD117	−	May be positive (about a third of cases)
CD27	+	71–81% + (more weakly expressed than in normal plasma cells)
CD28	−	+ in a third to a quarter of patients
CD81	+	− or weak
CD200	−	60–75% +
MUM1/IRF4	+	+
Antigen detected by VS38c	+	+
MYC	−	Sometimes +
Cyclin D1	−	Sometimes +, particularly but not only with t(11;14)
Cytoplasmic immunoglobulin	Polytypic (κ and λ)	Monotypic (κ or λ)

* CD79a, CD43 and MUM1/IRF4 are expressed in both; CD22 and surface membrane immunoglobulin are usually not expressed in either.

chains [78]. CD33 is aberrantly expressed in about a fifth of patients and is prognostically adverse. Lack of CD56 expression is also prognostically adverse [79]. CD38 expression may be lost for some months after daratumumab therapy. It should be noted that flow cytometry of an aspirate (and, similarly, bone marrow films) can underestimate the number of myeloma cells in comparison with immunohistochemistry on trephine biopsy or clot sections, there being on average 15% difference in one study [80]; when there is any discrepancy, it is the latter that should be relied on.

Plasma Cell Leukaemia

The immunophenotype of plasma cell leukaemia is similar to that of multiple myeloma with CD38, CD138 and cIg being positive and CD19, CD22 and CD45 being negative. CD20 has been reported as positive in 0–56% in four series of patients [81, 82]. CD56 is expressed less often than in multiple myeloma, being seen in four of nine cases in one study [81] and in 60% of 36 cases in another [82]. CD117 is expressed in about a quarter of patients [82].

Light Chain-associated Amyloidosis

Immunophenotyping is not useful in making this diagnosis. However, the presence of clonal plasma cells [83] or more than 2.5% clonal plasma cells [84] in the peripheral blood has been found to have an adverse prognostic significance in light chain-associated amyloidosis, significance being retained on multivariate analysis that includes the presence of at least 10% clonal plasma cells in the bone marrow [83].

Hodgkin Lymphoma

It is sometimes possible to diagnose Hodgkin lymphoma by flow cytometric immunophenotyping of a lymph node aspirate but this is not recommended since histology is important in making a precise diagnosis. However, immunohistochemistry to identify the characteristic immunophenotype of the neoplastic cells (Table 3.12) is of considerable importance.

Hodgkin/Reed–Sternberg cells in classical Hodgkin lymphoma express CD15 (70–80% of cases) and CD30 and also CD40, CD71, CD80, CD86, CD95, CD123, CD274 (PD-L1) and weak PAX5 [85–87]. EBV-related cases (20–25% of cases in developed countries, 70–90% in sub-Saharan Africa) show expression of LMP1, LMP2A and EBNA [88].

The neoplastic cells of nodular lymphocyte predominant Hodgkin lymphoma, however, have a clear-cut mature B-cell immunophenotype, express strong CD20 and EMA (CD227) and rarely express CD15 or CD30; they are designated LP cells and appear in a background of mature small B cells and with a meshwork of follicular T helper cells expressing CD4, CD57 and CD279 (PD-1). There is only very rarely a relationship to EBV infection [86].

The role of immunohistochemistry in the differential diagnosis of classical Hodgkin lymphoma is discussed by Wang *et al.* [86].

Mature T-lineage and NK-lineage Neoplasms

Immunophenotyping is important in the diagnosis of lymphomas of mature T and NK cells and in distinguishing them from precursor neoplasms. Sometimes the immunophenotype is sufficiently distinctive that a specific diagnosis is indicated, as in T-prolymphocytic leukaemia (T-PLL), adult T-cell leukaemia/lymphoma, hepatosplenic T-cell lymphoma, T-cell large granular lymphocytic leukaemia and ALK-positive anaplastic large cell lymphoma. Most mature T-cell neoplasms express CD4, an exception being T-cell large granular lymphocytic leukaemia, which expresses CD8. Most mature T-cell lymphomas express T-cell receptor (TCR) $\alpha\beta$, an exception being hepatosplenic T-cell lymphoma, which expresses TCR $\gamma\delta$. Table 3.13 [40]

Table 3.12 A comparison of the typical immunophenotype of neoplastic cells in classic and nodular lymphocyte predominant Hodgkin lymphoma [85–87].

	Classical Hodgkin lymphoma (Reed–Sternberg and mononuclear Hodgkin cells)	Nodular lymphocyte predominant Hodgkin lymphoma (LP cells)
CD15	+ (75–85%)	–
CD30	+	–
CD45	–	+
CD19	–	+ or –
CD20	– or, in a minority, + (generally weak)	+
CD79a	– or weak	+
PAX5	+ (weaker than on normal B cells)	+
OCT1, OCT2	– (in 90% of cases)	+
BOB1	– (in 90% of cases)	+
BCL2	+	–
BCL6	–	+
PU.1	–	+
MUM1/IRF4	+	usually –
EMA (CD227)	–	+ (more than 50% of cases)
PD-L1 (CD274)	+	–
EBV LMP1 and EBNA1	+ in a significant minority*	– (very rarely +)

* Depending on subtype and epidemiology
EBNA, Epstein–Barr virus nuclear antigen 1; EBV LMP1, Epstein–Barr virus latent membrane protein 1; EMA, epithelial membrane antigen.
Source: from refs. [85–87].

shows a panel of antibodies that can be used to characterise these neoplasms.

In addition to immunophenotyping for diagnostic purposes, the availability of the CD30 antibody–drug conjugate, brentuximab vedotin, is an indication to test for expression of the antigen in T-cell lymphomas in which it may be expressed, not only ALK-positive and ALK-negative anaplastic large T-cell lymphomas but also primary cutaneous anaplastic large cell lymphoma, peripheral T-cell lymphoma, not otherwise specified, lymphomatoid papulosis and transformed mycosis fungoides.

T-cell Prolymphocytic Leukaemia

The frequent expression of CD7 is useful in distinguishing T-PLL from other neoplasms of mature T cells, in which expression is uncommon. This condition is also unusual in that although the majority of cases are CD4+CD8–, about a quarter are CD4+CD8+ and a smaller minority are CD4–CD8+. SmCD3 may, in a small number of cases, be negative or weak; when negative, cCD3 may be expressed. There is expression of CD2, CD5 and CD7. Occasionally CD45 is negative [89]. CD26 is homogeneously expressed and CD52 is strongly expressed, this being relevant to therapy with alemtuzumab. Cytoplasmic TCL1 expression is demonstrable by flow cytometry and immunohistochemistry [90, 91]. Immunohistochemistry shows expression of S100 protein is in about a third of cases; it is not often positive in other T-cell lymphomas [90].

Table 3.13 Characteristic immunophenotype of mature T-cell and NK-cell neoplasms.

Marker	LGLL – T cell	CLPD – NK	T-PLL	ATLL	Sézary syndrome	AITL	ALK+ ALCL
CD2	++	++	++	++	++	++	+
CD3	++	−	+	++	++	+	−/+
CD5	−/+	−/+	++	++	++	++	−/+
CD7	−/+	−/+	++	−/+	−/+	−/+	−/+
CD4	−	−	++	++	++	++	+
CD8	++	−/+	−/+	−	−	−	−/+
CD16	++	++	−	−	−	−	−
CD25	−	−	−/+	++	−/+	−	++
CD56	−/+	+	−	−	−	−	−/+
CD57	++	+	−	−	−	−	−

The frequency with which a marker is positive in >30% of cells in a particular leukaemia is indicated as follows: ++, 80–100%, +, 40–80%; −/+, 10–40%; −, 0–9%.

ALK+ ALCL, ALK-positive anaplastic large cell lymphoma; AITL, angioimmunoblastic T-cell lymphoma; ATLL, adult T-cell leukaemia/lymphoma; CLPD – NK, chronic lymphoproliferative disorder of natural killer (NK) cells; LGLL, large granular lymphocytic leukaemia; T-PLL, T-cell prolymphocytic leukaemia.

Adult T-cell Leukaemia/Lymphoma

The frequent but not invariable expression of CD25 is useful in the diagnosis of adult T-cell leukaemia/lymphoma. A minority of cases are CD4-negative/CD8 positive or co-express CD4 and CD8. CD38, CD71 and HLA-DR are often expressed. CD30 may be expressed by larger cells. Expression of CD26 is weaker than expression by normal T cells.

Angioimmunoblastic T-cell Lymphoma

CD10, CD279 (PD-1) and BCL6, which are expressed by normal follicular helper T cells, are useful in the diagnosis of angioimmunoblastic T-cell lymphoma and other lymphomas of T-helper origin. In one large series of patients there was expression of CD3, CD4, CD5, CD7 (55% of cases), CD10 (43% of cases) and CD279 [92]. There is also often expression of CD2, CXCL1, CXCL13, CXCR5 and ICOS. The presence of a population of SmCD3− CD4+

lymphocytes in the peripheral blood has been found to be diagnostically useful, being observed in all 17 patients in one study [93]. Atypical B cells resembling Reed–Sternberg cells can be present [94].

Hepatosplenic T-cell Lymphoma

Hepatosplenic T-cell lymphoma usually shows expression of CD2, CD3 and TCRγδ with no expression of CD4, CD5 or TCRαβ. In a minority of cases there is expression of TCRαβ rather than TCRγδ. There is variable expression of CD7, CD8, CD11c, CD16 and CD56 while CD57 is negative. TIA-1 and granzyme M are expressed but not granzyme B or perforin. There can be expression of two or three of CD158a, b and e.

Primary Cutaneous γδ T-cell Lymphoma

Primary cutaneous γδ T-cell lymphoma usually shows expression of CD2, CD3, CD56,

TCRγδ and cytotoxic markers (granzyme B, perforin and TIA-1) with no expression of CD4 and variable expression of CD8 [95].

Anaplastic Large Cell Lymphomas

ALK-positive anaplastic large cell lymphoma, by definition, expresses ALK (CD246) and often CD25 (strongly), CD26, CD43, CD71, HLA-DR, EMA (CD227) and one or more of the cytotoxic granule proteins (TIA-1, granzyme B and perforin). CD30 is strongly expressed by larger cells. PD-L1 (CD274) is strongly expressed [96]. CD3 is negative in more than three quarters of cases. CD2, CD4 and CD5 are more often expressed. CD7 may be expressed [95]. On immuno-histochemistry, the location of ALK expression differs between cases with t(2;5) and those with variant translocations, and also between larger and smaller cells and between typical cases and the small cell variant [97]. MUM1/IRF4 may be expressed [98].

ALK-negative anaplastic large cell lymphoma, by definition, does not express CD246. As for ALK-positive cases, there is expression of CD43 and variable expression of other T-cell markers (CD2, CD3, CD4) and cytotoxic granule proteins. Expression of CD30 is uniform and strong. EMA (CD227) is often expressed (about 40% of cases). MUM1/IRF4 may be expressed [98].

Breast-implant-associated anaplastic lymphoma is ALK negative [99]. There is strong uniform expression of CD30. CD4 is often expressed while CD3 and CD5 are often negative.

Primary cutaneous anaplastic large cell lymphoma shows expression of CD4 and CD30 with variable loss of CD2, CD3 and CD5 [98, 100]. Only occasional cases are ALK positive [100]. Activation markers, such as CD25, CD71 and HLA-DR, and cytotoxic T-cell markers (granzyme B, TIA-1 and perforin) are expressed in some cases [100]. MUM1/IRF4 may be expressed [98].

Lymphomatoid Papulosis

Most cases are CD4+ CD8− with a minority being CD4− CD8+; CD2 and CD3 are expressed but CD7 expression is lost; CD30 is expressed [100]; some cases express CD56 or cytotoxic granule proteins [98]. Clinical and immunophenotypic features overlap with those of primary cutaneous anaplastic large cell lymphoma so that assessment of clinical presentation and observation for disease progression may be needed to make a distinction [101].

Sézary Syndrome

In addition to the immunophenotypic markers shown in Table 3.13, Sézary syndrome shows expression of CD279 (PD-1) and CD158k (or less often CD158a or CD158b) but not of CD26, an antigen expressed by activated T cells. Expression of CD2, CD3, CD4, CD5 or, most often, CD7 may be lost [102]. A CD4+ CD26− phenotype is useful in distinguishing cells of this syndrome from those of an inflammatory erythroderma. Diagnostic criteria used include CD4:CD8 ≥10, CD4+CD7− ≥ 30% and CD4+CD26− ≥40% [101].

Mycosis Fungoides

Mycosis fungoides usually shows expression of CD2, CD3, CD4, CD5 and CD45RO but expression of CD2, CD3 and CD5 may be lost [102]. There is usually no expression of CD7, CD8 or CD26 while expression of CD25 and CD30 is variable, correlating with transformation. Cytotoxic granule contents, TIA-1 and granzyme B are expressed in a minority of cases [102]. CD279 (PD-1) is often expressed.

Intestinal T-cell Lymphomas

There are differences in immunophenotype between intestinal lymphomas that are associated with coeliac disease and those that are not.

Enteropathy-associated T-cell lymphoma usually shows expression of CD2, CD3, CD7,

CD103 and cytotoxic granule proteins, TIA-1, granzyme B and perforin. CD4, CD5, TCRβ, TCRγ, CD16 and CD56 are not expressed. CD8 is expressed in a minority of patients. If larger cells are present, they are usually CD30 positive.

Cases of intestinal lymphoma now designated monomorphic intestinal epitheliotropic T-cell lymphoma show expression of CD3, CD8 and CD56 and often TCRγ. TIA-1 may be expressed. Other cytotoxic granule proteins and CD5 are negative [95]. CD103 and CD20 may be expressed [103].

T-cell Large Granular Lymphocytic Leukaemia

There is expression of CD2, CD3, CD8, CD16, CD57, TCRαβ and cytotoxic granule proteins, perforin, TIA-1, granzyme B and granzyme M; CD94 and CD161 are often expressed [104]. CD56 is usually negative. There is restricted or absent expression of CD158 epitopes, which provides indirect evidence of clonality.

Chronic Lymphoproliferative Disorder of NK Cells

This condition is negative for SmCD3, but immunohistochemistry may show positivity as a result of the presence of cytoplasmic CD3ε. There is expression of CD2, CD8, CD16, CD57 (weak), CD94 and cytotoxic granule proteins (TIA-1, granzyme B, granzyme M and perforin). CD56 is expressed in a minority of patients. Expression of only one epitope of CD158 (KIR receptor) – CD158a, CD158b or CD158e – or absent expression can provide surrogate evidence of clonality and thus permit neoplasia to be inferred.

Aggressive NK-cell Leukaemia

This lymphoma shows expression of CD2, usually CD16, CD56, CD94 and HLA-DR and is usually CD5, CD7 and CD57 negative [95]. SmCD3

is negative while, on immunohistochemistry, cytoplasmic CD3ε is positive. Cytotoxic granule proteins are expressed and CD7 may be expressed.

Extranodal NK/T-cell Lymphoma, Nasal Type

This lymphoma shows expression of CD2, CD56, perforin, granzyme B and TIA-1; CD25 and CD43 are often expressed and sometimes CD7. CD5 is usually negative [95]. CD3 is negative in NK lineage cases, but immunohistochemistry may show expression of cytoplasmic CD3ε. CD30 is positive in about a third of cases. EBV LMP1 is sometimes detectable on immunohistochemistry, but in *situ* hybridisation for EBER is the preferred technique and can permit identification of the uncommon examples of bone marrow infiltration. There is expression of PD-L1 (CD274) and responsiveness to treatment with the PD-1 (CD279) antibody, pembrolizumab [105].

T-lineage cases may express CD5 and CD8 as well as TCR αβ or γδ.

Systemic EBV-positive T-cell Lymphoma of Childhood

Lymphoma cells usually express CD2, CD3 and TIA-1 with CD56 being negative. Cases occurring in the setting of acute EBV infection tend to be CD8 positive while those in the setting of chronic active EBV infection are CD4 positive.

Minimal Residual Disease

Table 3.14 shows markers that can be applied for the detection of minimal residual disease (or more correctly 'measurable residual disease') [77, 106–115]. This can be based on: (i) under-expression; (ii) over-expression; (iii) aberrant expression; or (iv) asynchronous expression of antigens. It is possible either to

Table 3.14 Antibodies that can be used in panels for monitoring minimal residual disease*.

Disease	Applicable antibodies
B-lineage acute lymphoblastic leukaemia (B-ALL) [107]	UK Flow MRD Working Group panel: CD38, CD45, CD58 and CD123 (backbone CD10, CD19 and CD34)
	EuroFlow panel: CD73, CD66c, CD81, CD304 (backbone CD10, CD19, CD20, CD34, CD45) [108]
	Children's Oncology Group panel: CD9, CD10, CD19, CD20, CD13, CD33, CD34, CD38, CD45, CD58 and SYTO-16 (to identify all nucleated cells) [109]
	Also applicable: CD11a, CD11b, CD15, CD21, CD22, CD24, CD25, CD44, CD49b, CD49f, CD65, CD72, CD79b, CD86, CD97, CD99, CD102, CD164, CD200, CD304, CD371, NG2, TdT and HLA-DR
T-lineage acute lymphoblastic leukaemia (T-ALL)	UK Flow MRD Working Group panel: CD1a, CD2, cCD3, CD4, CD5, CD8, CD10, CD13, CD33, CD34, CD38, CD56, CD99, TdT and HLA-DR (backbone FSC, SSC, CD7, SmCD3)
	Children's Oncology Group panel: (replace CD48 for CD2) [109]
	Also applicable: mCD3, CD7, CD11b, CD16, CD45, CD117 and CD335
Acute myeloid leukaemia (AML)	European LeukemiaNet panel: CD7, CD11b, CD13, CD15, CD19, CD33, CD34, CD45, CD56, CD117, HLA-DR (backbone: CD45, CD34, CD117, CD13, CD33, FSC/SSC); if necessary, supplement with a 'monocyte tube' – CD64/CD11b/CD14/CD4/CD34/HLA-DR/CD33/CD45 [110]
	Also applicable: CD2, CD5, CD10, CD16, CD19, CD20, CD22, CD38, CD41, CD61, CD65, CD71, CD123, CD133, CD235a, TdT and MPO
Chronic lymphocytic leukaemia (CLL)	ERIC (European Research Initiative on CLL) panel: CD5 (+), CD19 (+), CD20 (weak), CD43 (stronger than normal B cells), CD79b (weak or –), CD81 (weak or –) and SSC; CD22 (weak or –) is an important addition shortly after anti-CD20 therapy [111, 112]
	Also applicable CD23, CD30, CD38, CD160, CD200 and ROR1 [111–113]
Hairy cell leukaemia	CD11c, CD19, CD20, CD22, CD25, CD45, CD103, CD123, CD200 and CD305 (and high SSC) [114]
Multiple myeloma	EuroFlow panel: CD19, CD27, CD38, CD45, CD56, CD81, CD117, CD138, cκ and cλ [77]
	Also applicable: CD20, CD28, CD200, CD229, cκ and cλ) [77, 115]

Abbreviations: c, cytoplasmic; FSC, forward scatter; MPO, myeloperoxidase; Sm, surface membrane; SSC, sideways scatter; TdT, terminal deoxynucleotidyl transferase.
* Some antibodies are included in panels for gating purposes and others for the demonstration of an abnormal phenotype

define a leukaemia-associated immunophenotype at diagnosis or to look for immunophenotypic divergence from what is expected in normal or regenerating bone marrow, the latter policy avoiding problems due to immunophenotypic shift occurring during the course of a disease. Multicolour flow cytometry is needed so that the expression of individual antigens of interest can be assessed on a backbone defined by core antigens.

Acute Lymphoblastic Leukaemia

In B-ALL, it is necessary to distinguish between residual leukaemic lymphoblasts and normal regenerating B-cell precursors (haematogones) (see earlier); this is dependent on aberrant expression (e.g. of CD13, CD15, CD33, CD56, CD117), on the over- or under-expression of antigens by leukaemic lymphoblasts and on the more heterogeneous expression of antigens by haematogones in comparison with lymphoblasts. CD66c expression is particularly useful for Ph-positive and high hyperdiploid B-ALL and CD123 expression is also associated with high hyperdiploid ALL [116]. NG2 and CD15 can be expressed in *KMT2A*-rearranged ALL.

In the case of T-ALL, detection of antigens that are normally only expressed by thymic cells is important as well as aberrant antigen expression (e.g. of CD11b, CD13, CD33, CD117 and CD335). Expression of CD10, CD34, CD99 and TdT may decline during therapy [117].

In B- and T-ALL, it has been found that flow cytometric evidence of 5% or more blast cells in patients who are assessed as being in morphological remission is prognostically adverse and it is suggested that they should not be regarded as being in complete remission [109].

Acute Myeloid Leukaemia

In AML, detection of MRD is dependent of under- and over-expression of antigens, asynchronous expression and aberrant expression.

Chronic Lymphocytic Leukaemia

The detection of MRD during and following therapy for CLL carries prognostic significance. MRD negativity, defined as less than one CLL cell in 10,000 in blood or bone marrow, is associated with a longer progression-free survival and treatment-free interval. Although clinical decision making is not currently using MRD data, it is being assessed in ongoing clinical trials and it is likely that such MRD-based response assessments will guide patient management in the future.

B-lineage Non-Hodgkin Lymphoma

MRD is predictive of progression-free survival in follicular lymphoma.

Hairy Cell Leukaemia

Detection of MRD in hairy cell leukaemia is straightforward but its significance is controversial since some years may pass before further therapy is needed [114].

Multiple Myeloma

In multiple myeloma, CD19, CD38, CD45 and CD56 provide a suitable panel in more than 90% of patients. PD-1 (CD279) and PD-L1 (CD274) may be upregulated when there is MRD [45].

Paroxysmal Nocturnal Haemoglobinuria

The immunophenotypic diagnosis of PNH depends on the detection of either (i) absent or reduced expression of antigens that are bound to membrane glycosylphosphatidylinositol (GPI) or (ii) reduction of membrane GPI by showing reduced binding of fluorescent aerolysin (FLAER). Table 3.15 shows applicable markers [118]. For each lineage studied, two antibodies or one antibody and FLAER should be used. Rather confusingly, cells with a total deficiency are referred to as type III cells and those with a partial deficiency as type II cells (type I being normal).

Non-haematological Tumours

Non-haematological tumours infiltrating the bone marrow can be investigated by flow cytometry or immunohistochemistry. The small cell tumours of childhood enter into the differential diagnosis of ALL and may be recognised on flow cytometry. Carcinomas and sarcomas are usually investigated by immunohistochemistry on trephine biopsy sections [119]. Immunohistochemical markers for carcinoma include various cytokeratins, CD227 (epithelial membrane antigen) and carcinoembryonic antigen (CD66e). Specific types of carcinoma, for example, carcinoma of the prostate, breast, thyroid, and ovary or endometrium, can also be recognised with specific antibodies [119]. Vascular tumours can be recognised by expression of CD31, CD34, CD117, FLI1, ERG and von Willebrand factor. Melanoma

Table 3.15 Markers that can be used in the flow cytometric diagnosis of paroxysmal nocturnal haemoglobinuria.

Lineage being studied	Marker to identify lineage	FLAER and applicable antibodies
Neutrophil	SSC and CD15 (or FSC, CD33 or CD45)	FLAER and CD24 or CD16* (or CD15, CD55, CD59, CD66, CD87 or CD157)
Monocyte	SSC and CD64 (or CD4 or CD33)	FLAER and CD14 (or CD52, CD55, CD64 or CD157)
Erythrocyte	FSC and CD235a	CD55 and CD59

Abbreviations: FSC, forward scatter; FLAER, fluorescent aerolysin; SSC side scatter.
* Expression of CD16 on NK cells is normal

shows expression of MelanA, MUM1/IRF4 and the antigen recognised by HMB-45.

Conclusion

Flow cytometric immunophenotyping and immunohistochemistry have greatly enhanced our ability to make a precise diagnosis in haematological disorders. However, considerable technical expertise and detailed knowledge are required, with all data being interpreted in the context of the clinical features and the cytological/histological characteristics of the cells and tissues studied.

References

1 Jaffe ES, Campo E, Harris NL, Pileri SA and Swerdlow SH (2017) Introduction and overview of the classification of lymphoid neoplasms, In: Swerdlow SH, Campo E, Harris NL, Jaffe ES, Pileri S, Stein H and Thiele J (eds) *WHO Classification of Tumours of Haematopoietic and Lymphoid Tissues*, revised 4th edn. IARC Press, Lyon, pp. 190–198.

2 Döhner H, Estey E, Grimwade D, Amadori S, Appelbaum FR, Büchner T *et al.* (2017) Diagnosis and management of AML in adults: 2017 ELN recommendations from an international expert panel. *Blood*, 129, 424–447.

3 Tiribelli M, Raspadori D, Geromin A, Cavallin M, Sirianni S, Simeone E *et al.* (2017) High CD200 expression is associated with poor prognosis in cytogenetically normal acute myeloid leukemia, even in FlT3-ITD-/NPM1+ patients. *Leuk Res*, 58, 31–38.

4 Klairmont MM, Hoskoppal D, Yadak N and Choi JK (2018) The comparative sensitivity of immunohistochemical markers of megakaryocytic differentiation in acute megakaryoblastic leukemia. *Am J Clin Pathol*, 150, 461–467.

5 Bain BJ and Béné MC (2019) Morphological and immunophenotypic clues to the WHO categories of acute myeloid leukaemia. *Acta Haematologica*, 141, 232–244.

6 Ren F, Zhang N, Xu Z, Xu J, Zhang Y, Chen X *et al.* (2019) The CD9+CD11b−HLA-DR− immunophenotype can be used to diagnose acute promyelocytic leukemia. *Int J Lab Haematol*, 41, 158–175.

7 Sobas M, Montesinos P, Boluda B, Bernal T, Vellenga E, Nomdedeu J *et al.*; PETHEMA, HOVON, PALG, and GATLA cooperative groups (2019) An analysis of the impact of CD56 expression in de novo acute promyelocytic leukemia patients treated with upfront all-trans retinoic acid and

anthracycline-based regimens. *Leuk Lymphoma*, 60, 1030–1035.

8 Patel SS, Pinkus GS, Ritterhouse LL, Segak JP, Cin PD, Restrepo T *et al.* (2019) High *NPM1* mutant allele burden at diagnosis correlates with minimal residual disease at first remission in de novo acute myeloid leukemia. *Am J Hematol*, 94, 921–928.

9 Mannelli F, Ponziani V, Bencini S, Bonetti MI, Benelli M, Cutini I *et al.* (2017) CEBPA-double-mutated acute myeloid leukemia displays a unique phenotypic profile: a reliable screening method and insight into biological features. *Haematologica*, 102, 529–540.

10 Marcolin R, Guolo F, Minetto P, Clavio M, Ballerini F, Manconi L *et al.* (2019) A simple cytofluorometric score may optimize testing for biallelic CEBPA mutations in patients with acute myeloid leukemia. *Haematologica*, 104, S2, 137.

11 Tang JL, Hou HA, Chen CY, Liu CY, Chou WC, Tseng MH *et al.* (2009) AML1/RUNX1 mutations in 470 adult patients with de novo acute myeloid leukemia: Prognostic implication and interaction with other gene alterations. *Blood*, 114, 5352–5361.

12 Tunstall O, Bhatnagar N, James B, Norton A, O'Marcaigh AS, Greenough A *et al.* (2018) Guidelines for the investigation and management of transient leukaemia of Down syndrome, *Br J Haematol*, 182, 200–211.

13 Karandikar NJ, Aquino DB, McKenna RW and Kroft SH (2001) Transient myeloproliferative disorder and acute myeloid leukemia in Down syndrome. An immunophenotypic analysis. *Am J Clin Pathol*, 116, 204–210.

14 Bride KL, Vincent TL, Im SY, Aplenc R, Barrett DM, Carroll WL *et al.* (2018) Preclinical efficacy of daratumumab in T-cell acute lymphoblastic leukemia. *Blood*, 131, 995–999.

15 Pileri SA, Ascano S, Milani M, Visani G, Piccioli M, Orcioni CF *et al.* (1999) Acute leukaemia immunophenotyping in bone-marrow routine sections. *Br J Haematol*, 105, 394–401.

16 Hashimoto M, Yamashita Y and Mori N (2002) Immunohistochemical detection of CD79a expression in precursor T cell lymphoblastic lymphoma/leukaemias. *J Pathol*, 197, 341–347.

17 Kansal R, Deeb G, Barcos M, Wetzler M, Brecher ML, Block AW and Stewart CC (2004) Precursor B lymphoblastic leukemia with surface light chain immunoglobulin restriction: A report of 15 patients. *Am J Clin Pathol*, 121, 512–525.

18 Guillaume N, Penther D, Vaida I, Gruson B, Harrivel V, Claisse JF *et al.* (2011) CD66c expression in B-cell acute lymphoblastic leukemia: Strength and weakness. *Int J Lab Hematol*, 33, 92–96.

19 Tsagarakis NJ, Papadhimitriou SI, Pavlidis D, Marinakis T, Kostopoulos IV, Stiakaki E *et al.* (2019) Flow cytometric predictive scoring systems for common fusions ETV6/RUNX1, BCR/ABL1, TCF3/PBX1 and rearrangements of the KMT2A gene, proposed for the initial cytogenetic approach in cases of B-acute lymphoblastic leukemia. *Int J Lab Hematol*, 41, 364–372.

20 Borowitz MJ, Chan JKC, Béné MC and Arber DA (2017) T lymphoblastic leukaemia/lymphoma, In: Swerdlow SH, Campo E, Harris NL, Jaffe ES, Pileri S, Stein H and Thiele J (eds) *WHO Classification of Tumours of Haematopoietic and Lymphoid Tissues*, revised 4th edn. IARC Press, Lyon, pp. 209–212.

21 Krogeer H, Rahman H, Jain N, Angelova EA, Yang H, Quesada A *et al.* (2019) Early T precursor acute lymphoblastic leukaemia/lymphoma shows differential immunophenotypic characteristics including frequent CD33 expression and *in vitro* response to targeted CD33 therapy. *Br J Haematol*, 186, 538–548.

22 Boddu P, Thakral B, Alhuraiji A, Pemmaraju N, Kadia T, Ohanian M *et al.* (2019) Distinguishing thymoma from T-lymphoblastic leukaemia/lymphoma: a

case-based evaluation. *J Clin Pathol*, 72, 251–257.

23 Borowitz MJ, Béné MC, Harris NL, Porwit A, Matutes E and Arber DA (2017) Acute leukaemias of ambiguous lineage, In: Swerdlow SH, Campo E, Harris NL, Jaffe ES, Pileri S, Stein H and Thiele J (eds) *WHO Classification of Tumours of Haematopoietic and Lymphoid Tissues*, revised 4th edn. IARC Press, Lyon, pp. 209–212.

24 Ogata K, Kishikawa Y, Satoh C, Tamura H, Dan K and Hayashi A (2006) Diagnostic application of flow cytometric characteristics of CD34$^+$ cells in low-grade myelodysplastic syndromes *Blood*, 108, 1037–1044.

25 Della Porta MG, Picone C, Pascutto C, Malcovati L, Tamura H, Handa H *et al.* (2012) Multicenter validation of a reproducible flow cytometric score for the diagnosis of low-grade myelodysplastic syndromes: Results of a European LeukemiaNET study. *Haematologica*, 97, 1209–1217.

26 Montauban SG, Hernandez-Perez CR, Veloso EDRP, Novoa V, Lorand-Metz I, Gonzalez J *et al.* (2019) Flow cytometry "Ogata score" for the diagnosis of myelodysplastic syndromes in a real-life setting. A Latin American experience. *Int J Lab Hematol*, 41, 536–541.

27 Selimoglu-Buet D, Wagner-Ballon O, Saada V, Bardet V, Itzykson R, Bencheikh L *et al.*; Francophone Myelodysplasia Group (2015) Characteristic repartition of monocyte subsets as a diagnostic signature of chronic myelomonocytic leukemia. *Blood*, 125, 3618–3626.

28 Itzykson R, Fenaux P, Bowen D, Cross NCP, Cortes J, De Witte T *et al.* (2018) Diagnosis and treatment of chronic myelomonocytic leukemias in adults: recommendations from the European Hematology Association and the European LeukemiaNet. *Hemasphere*, 2, e150.

29 Hudson CA, Burack WR and Bennett JM (2018) Emerging utility of flow cytometry in the diagnosis of chronic myelomonocytic leukemia. *Leuk Res*, 73, 12–15.

30 Chen JX, Mei LP, Chen BG, Wang DL, Luo WD, Luo LF *et al.* (2017) Over-expression of CD200 predicts poor prognosis in MDS. *Leuk Res*, 56, 1–6.

31 Moonin MT, Kossier T, van de Walt J, Wilkins B, Harrison CN and Radhia DH (2012) CD30/CD123 expression in systemic mastocytosis does not correlate with aggressive disease. *Blood*, 120, 1746.

32 Pardanani A, Reichard KK, Zblewski D, Abdelrahman RA, Wassie EA, Morice WG *et al.* (2016) CD123 immunostaining patterns in systemic mastocytosis: differential expression in disease subgroups and potential prognostic value. *Leukemia*, 30, 914–918.

33 Perbellini O, Zamò A, Colarossi S, Zampieri F, Zoppi F, Bonadonna P *et al.* (2011) Primary role of multiparametric flow cytometry in the diagnostic work-up of indolent clonal mast cell disorders. *Cytometry Part B*, 80B, 362–368.

34 Bosch-Vilaseca A, Monter-Rovira A, Cisa-Wieczorek S, Oñate G, Bussaglia E, Carricondo M *et al.* (2019) Ultrastructural, cytogenetic, and molecular findings in mast cell leukemia: Case report. *Clin Case Rep*, 7, 1395–1398.

35 Mannelli F, Gesullo F, Rotunno G, Pacilli A, Bencini S, Annunziato F *et al.* (2019) Myelodysplasia as assessed by multiparameter flow cytometry refines prognostic stratification provided by genotypic risk in systemic mastocytosis. *Am J Hematol*, 94, 845–852.

36 Taylor J, Haddadin M, Upadhyay VA, Grussie E, Mehta-Shah N, Brunner AM *et al.* (2019) Multicenter analysis of outcomes in blastic plasmacytoid dendritic cell neoplasm offers a pretargeted therapy benchmark. *Blood*, 134, 678–687.

37 Facchetti F, Lonardi S, Vermi W and Lorenzi L (2019) Updates in histiocytic and dendritic cell proliferations and neoplasms. *Diagnostic Histopathol*, 25, 217–228.

38 Geissmann F, Lepelletier Y, Fraitag S, Valladeau J, Bodemer C, Debré M *et al.*

(2001) Differentiation of Langerhans cells in Langerhans cell histiocytosis. *Blood*, 97, 1241–1248.

39 Pillai V, Pozdnyakova O, Charest K, Li B, Shahsafaei A and Dorfman DM (2013) CD200 flow cytometric assessment and semiquantitative immunohistochemical staining distinguishes hairy cell leukemia from hairy cell leukemia-variant and other B-cell lymphoproliferative disorders. *Am J Clin Pathol*, 140, 536–543.

40 Bain BJ (2017) *Leukaemia Diagnosis*, 5th edn. Wiley Blackwell, Oxford, pp. 417–524.

41 Choi SM, Betz BL and Perry AM (2018) Follicular lymphoma diagnostic caveats and updates. *Arch Pathol Lab Med*, 142, 1330–1340.

42 D'Arena G, Vitale C, Rossi G, Coscia M, Omedè P, D'Auria F *et al.* (2018) CD200 included in a 4-marker modified Matutes score provides optimal sensitivity and specificity for the diagnosis of chronic lymphocytic leukaemia. *Hematol Oncol*, 35, 543–546.

43 Matutes E, Owusu-Ankomah K, Morilla R, Garcia-Marco J, Houlihan A, Que TH and Catovsky D (1994) The immunological profile of B-cell disorders and proposal of a scoring system for the diagnosis of CLL. *Leukemia*, 8, 1640–1645.

44 Köhnke T, Wittmann VK, Bücklein VL, Lichtenegger F, Pasalic Z, Hiddemann W *et al.* (2017) Diagnosis of CLL revisited: increased specificity by a modified five-marker scoring system including CD200. *Br J Haematol*, 179, 480–487.

45 Annibali O, Crescenzi A, Tomarchio V, Pagano A, Bianchi A, Grifoni A and Avvisati G (2018) PD-1 /PD-L1 checkpoint in hematological malignancies. *Leuk Res*, 67, 45–55.

46 Domingo A, Gonzáles-Barca E, Castellsagué X, Fernandez-Sevilla A, Graňema A, Crespo N and Ferrán C (1997) Expression of adhesion molecules in 113 patients with B-cell chronic lymphocytic leukemia: relationship with clinico-prognostic feature. *Leuk Res*, 21, 67–73.

47 Hjalmar V, Hast R and Kimby E (2002) Cell surface expression of CD25, CD54, and CD95 on B- and T-cells in chronic lymphocytic leukaemia in relation to trisomy 12, atypical morphology and clinical course. *Eur J Haematol*, 68, 127–134.

48 Rawstron AC, Kreuzer KA, Soosapilla A, Spacek M, Stehlikova O, Gambell P *et al.* (2018) Reproducible diagnosis of chronic lymphocytic leukemia by flow cytometry: An European Research Initiative on CLL (ERIC) & European Society for Clinical Cell Analysis (ESCCA) Harmonisation project. *Cytometry B Clin Cytom*, 94, 121–128.

49 Friedman DR, Guadalupe E, Volkheimer A, Moore JO and Weinberg JB (2018) Clinical outcomes in chronic lymphocytic leukaemia associated with expression of CD5, a negative regulator of B-cell receptor signalling. *Br J Haematol*, 183, 747–754.

50 Ito M, Iida S, Inagaki H, Tsuboi K, Komatsu H, Yamaguchi M *et al.* (2002) MUM1/IRF4 expression is an unfavorable prognostic factor in B-cell chronic lymphocytic leukemia (CLL)/small lymphocytic lymphoma (SLL). *Jpn J Cancer Res*, 93, 685–694.

51 McKay P, Leach M, Jackson B, Robinson S and Rule S (2018) A British Society for Haematology good practice paper on the diagnosis and investigation of patients with mantle cell lymphoma. *Br J Haematol*, 182, 63–70.

52 Liu Z, Dong HY, Gorczyca W, Tsang P, Cohen P, Stephenson CF *et al.* (2002) CD5− mantle cell lymphoma. *Am J Clin Pathol*, 118, 216–224.

53 Barna G, Mihalik R, Timár B, Tömböl J, Csende Z, Sebestyén A *et al.* (2011) ROR1 expression is not a unique marker of CLL. *Hematol Oncol*, 29, 17–21.

54 NordiQC Immunochemistry Quality Control. https://www.nordiqc.org/epitope. php?id=55

55 Mackrides N, Chapman J, Larson MC, Ramos JC, Toomey N, Lin P *et al.* (2019) Prevalence, clinical characteristics and

prognosis of EBV-positive follicular lymphoma. *Am J Hematol*, 94, E62–E64.

56 Kiesewetter B, Simonitsch-Klupp I, Kornauth C, Dolak W, Lukas J, Mayerhoefer ME and Raderer M (2018) Immunohistochemical expression of cereblon and MUM1 as potential predictive markers of response to lenalidomide in extranodal marginal zone B-cell lymphoma of the mucosa-associated lymphoid tissue (MALT lymphoma). *Hematol Oncol*, 36, 62–67.

57 Owen RG, Pratt G, Auer RL, Flatley R, Kyriakou C, Lunn MP *et al.*; British Committee for Standards in Haematology (2014) Guidelines on the diagnosis and management of Waldenström macroglobulinaemia. *Br J Haematol*, 165, 316–333.

58 Morice WG, Chen D, Kurtin PJ, Hanson CA and McPhail ED (2009) Novel immunophenotypic features of marrow lymphoplasmacytic lymphoma and correlation with Waldenström's macroglobulinemia. *Mod Pathol*, 22, 807–816.

59 Raimbault A, Machherndl-Spandl S, Itzykson R, Clauser S, Chapuis N, Mathis S *et al.* (2019) CD13 expression in B cell malignancies is a hallmark of plasmacytic differentiation. *Br J Haematol*, 184, 625–633.

60 Hiemcke-Jiwa LS, Leguit RJ, Jiwa NM, Huibers MMH and Minnema MC (2019) *CXCR4* mutations in lymphoplasmacytic lymphoma lead to altered CXCR4 expression. *Br J Haematol*, 185, 966–969.

61 Jones G, Parry-Jones N, Wilkins B, Else M and Catovsky D; British Committee for Standards in Haematology (2012) Revised guidelines for the diagnosis and management of hairy cell leukaemia and hairy cell leukaemia variant* (*sic*). *Br J Haematol*, 156, 186–195.

62 Matutes E, Martínez-Trillos A and Campo E (2015) Hairy cell leukaemia-variant: Disease features and treatment. *Best Pract Res Clin Haematol*, 28, 253–263.

63 Traverse-Glehen A, Baseggio L, Bauchu EC, Morel D, Gazzo S, French M *et al.* (2008) Splenic red pulp lymphoma with numerous basophilic villous lymphocytes: a distinct clinicopathologic and molecular entity? *Blood*, 111, 2253–2260.

64 Navid F, Mosijczuk AD, Head DR, Borowitz MJ, Carroll AJ, Brandt JM *et al.* (1999) Acute lymphoblastic leukemia with the (8,14) (q24;q32) translocation and FAB L3 morphology associated with a B-precursor immunophenotype: The Pediatric Oncology Group experience. *Leukemia*, 13, 135–141.

65 Hans CP, Weisenburger DD, Greiner TC, Gascoyne RD, Delabie J, Ott G *et al.* (2004) Confirmation of the molecular classification of diffuse large B-cell lymphoma by immunohistochemistry using a tissue microarray. *Blood*, 103, 275–282.

66 Visco C, Li Y, Xu-Monette ZY, Miranda RN, Green TM, Li Y *et al.* (2012) Comprehensive gene expression profiling and immunohistochemical studies support application of immunophenotypic algorithm for molecular subtype classification in diffuse large B-cell lymphoma: A report from the International DLBCL Rituximab-CHOP Consortium Program Study. *Leukemia*, 26, 2103–2113.

67 Bledsoe JR, Redd RA, Hasserjian RP, Soumerai JD, Nishino HT, Boyer DF *et al.* (2016) The immunophenotypic spectrum of primary mediastinal large B-cell lymphoma reveals prognostic biomarkers associated with outcome. *Am J Hematol*, 91, E436–E441.

68 Brimo F, Michel RP, Khetani K and Auger M (2007) Primary effusion lymphoma: A series of 4 cases and review of the literature with emphasis on cytomorphologic and immunocytochemical differential diagnosis. *Cancer Cytopathol*, 111, 224–233.

69 Oksenhendler E, Boutboul D and Galicier L (2019) Kaposi sarcoma-associated herpesvirus/human herpesvirus 8-associated lymphoproliferative disorders. *Blood*, 133, 1186–1190.

70 Mendeville M, Roemer MGM, van den Hout MFCM, Los-de Vries GT, Bladergroen R, Stathi P *et al.* (2019) Aggressive genomic features in clinically indolent primary HHV8-negative effusion-based lymphoma. *Blood*, 133, 377–380.

71 Geer M, Roberts E, Shango M, Till BG, Smith SD, Abbas H *et al.* (2019) Multicentre retrospective study of intravascular large B-cell lymphoma treated at academic institutions within the United States. *Br J Haematol*, 186, 255–262.

72 Kim WY, Puch M, Dojcinov S and Quintanilla-Martinez L (2019) 'Grey zones' in the differential diagnosis of lymphoma pathology. *Diagnostic Histopathology*, 25, 191–216.

73 Campo E, Stein H and Harris NL (2017) Plasmablastic lymphoma. In Swerdlow SH, Campo E, Harris NL, Jaffe ES, Pileri S, Stein H and Thiele J (eds) *WHO Classification of Tumours of Haematopoietic and Lymphoid Tissues*, revised 4th edn. IARC Press, Lyon, pp. 321–322.

74 Shi J, Bodo J, Zhao X, Durkin L, Goyal T, Meyerson H and Hsi ED (2019) SLAMF7 (CD319/CS1) is expressed in plasmablastic lymphoma and is a potential diagnostic marker and therapeutic target. *Br J Haematol*, 185, 145–147.

75 Paiva B, Gutiérrez NC, Chen X, Vidriales MB, Montalbán MA, Rosiñol L *et al.*; GEM (Grupo Español de Mieloma)/PETHEMA (Programa para el Estudio de la Terapéutica en Hemopatias Malignas) cooperative (2012) Clinical significance of CD81 expression by clonal plasma cells in high-risk smoldering and symptomatic multiple myeloma patients. *Leukemia*, 26, 1862–1869.

76 Tembhare PR, Yuan C, Korde N, Maric I, Calvo K, Yancey MA *et al.* (2011) Highly sensitive marker in flow cytometric diagnosis of plasma cell dyscrasia. *Blood*, 118, 2880.

77 Flores-Montero J, Sanoja-Flores L, Paiva B, Puig N, García-Sánchez O, Böttcher S *et al.* (2017) Next Generation Flow for highly sensitive and standardized detection of

minimal residual disease in multiple myeloma. *Leukemia*, 31, 2094–2103.

78 Kurt H and Ferreira KA (2019) Biphenotypic plasma cell myeloma. *Blood*, 133, 1611.

79 Skerget M, Skopec B, Zadnik V, Zontar D, Podgornik H, Rebersek K *et al.* (2018) CD56 expression is an important prognostic factor in multiple myeloma even with bortezomib induction. *Acta Haematol*, 139, 228–234.

80 Matsue K, Matsue Y, Kumata K, Usui Y, Suehara Y, Fukumoto K *et al.* (2017) Quantification of bone marrow plasma cell infiltration in multiple myeloma: usefulness of bone marrow aspirate clot with CD138 immunohistochemistry. *Hematol Oncol*, 35, 323–328.

81 Tembhare PR, Subramanian PG, Sehgal K, Yajamanam B, Kumar A, Gadge V *et al.* (2011) Immunophenotypic profile of plasma cell leukemia: A retrospective study in a reference cancer center in India and review of literature. *Indian J Pathol Microbiol*, 54, 294–298.

82 Kraj M, Kopeć-Szlęzak J, Pogłód R and Kruk B (2011) Flow cytometric immunophenotypic characteristics of plasma cell leukemia. *Folia Histochem Cytobiol*, 49, 168–182.

83 Sidana S, Tandon N, Dispenzieri A, Gertz MA, Dingli D, Jevremovic D *et al.* (2018) Prognostic significance of circulating plasma cells by multi-parametric flow cytometry in light chain amyloidosis. *Leukemia*, 32, 1421–1426.

84 Muchtar E, Jevremovic D, Dispenzieri A, Dingli D, Buadi FK, Lacy MQ *et al.* (2017) The prognostic value of multiparametric flow cytometry in AL amyloidosis at diagnosis and at the end of first-line treatment. *Blood*, 129, 82–87.

85 McKay P, Fielding P, Gallop-Evans E, Hall GW, Lambert J, Leach M *et al.*; British Committee for Standards in Haematology (2016) Guidelines for the investigation and management of nodular lymphocyte predominant Hodgkin lymphoma. *Br J Haematol*, 172, 32–43.

86 Wang HW, Balakrishna JP, Pittaluga S and Jaffe ES (2019) Diagnosis of Hodgkin lymphoma in the modern era. *Br J Haematol*, 184, 45–59.

87 Cirillo M, Reinke S, Klapper W and Borchmann S (2019) The translational science of hodgkin (*sic*) lymphoma. *Br J Haematol*, 184, 30–44.

88 Murray PG and Young LS (2019) An etiological role for the Epstein-Barr virus in the pathogenesis of classical Hodgkin lymphoma. *Blood*, 134, 591–596.

89 Thakral B and Wang SA (2018) T-cell prolymphocytic leukemia negative for surface CD3 and CD45. *Blood*, 132, 111.

90 Aggarwal N, Pongpruttipan T, Patel S, Bayerl MG, Alkan S, Nathwani B *et al.* (2015) Expression of S100 Protein in CD4-positive T-cell lymphomas is often associated with T-cell prolymphocytic leukemia. *Am J Surg Pathol*, 39, 1679–1687.

91 Staber PB, Herling M, Bellido M, Jacobsen ED, Davids MS, Kadia TM *et al.* (2019) Consensus criteria for diagnosis, staging, and treatment response assessment of T-cell prolymphocytic leukemia. *Blood*, 134, 1132–1143.

92 Hong H, Fang X, Wang Z, Huang H, Lam ST, Li F *et al.* (2018) Angioimmunoblastic T-cell lymphoma: a prognostic model from a retrospective study. *Leuk Lymphoma*, 59, 2911–2916.

93 Singh A, Schabath R, Ratei R, Stroux A, Klemke CD, Nebe T *et al.* (2014) Peripheral blood sCD3$^-$ CD4$^+$ T cells: A useful diagnostic tool in angioimmunoblastic T cell lymphoma. *Hematol Oncol*, 32, 16–21.

94 Kim WY, Pugh M, Dojcinov S and Quintanilla-Martinez L (2019) 'Grey zones' in the differential diagnosis of lymphoma pathology. *Diagn Histopathol*, 25, 191–216.

95 Zain JM (2019) Aggressive T-cell lymphomas: 2019 updates on diagnosis, risk stratification, and management. *Am J Hematol*, 94, 929–946.

96 Zhang JP, Song Z, Wang HB, Lang L, Yang YZ, Xiao W *et al.* (2019) A novel model of controlling PD-L1 expression in ALK$^+$ anaplastic large cell lymphoma revealed by CRISPR screening. *Blood*, 134, 171–185.

97 Falini B, Lamant-Rochaix L, Campo E, Jaffe ES, Gascoyne RD, Stein H *et al.* (2017) Anaplastic large cell lymphoma, ALK-positive, In: Swerdlow SH, Campo E, Harris NL, Jaffe ES, Pileri S, Stein H and Thiele J (eds) *WHO Classification of Tumours of Haematopoietic and Lymphoid Tissues*, revised 4th edn. IARC Press, Lyon, pp. 413−418.

98 Shinohara MM and Shustov A (2019) How I treat primary cutaneous CD30$^+$ lymphoproliferative disorders. *Blood*, 134, 515–524.

99 Mehta-Shah N, Clemens MW and Horwitz SM (2018) How I treat breast implant-associated anaplastic large cell lymphoma. *Blood*, 132, 1889–1898.

100 Prieto-Torres L, Rodriguez-Pinilla SM, Onaindia A, Ara M, Requena L and Piris MÁ (2019) CD30-positive primary cutaneous lymphoproliferative disorders: molecular alterations and targeted therapies. *Haematologica*, 104, 226–235.

101 Willemze R, Cerroni L, Kempf W, Berti E, Facchetti F, Swerdlow SH and Jaffe ES (2019) The 2018 update of the WHO-EORTC classification for primary cutaneous lymphomas. *Blood*, 133, 1703−1714.

102 Willemze R, Jaffe ES, Burg G, Cerroni L, Berti E, Swerdlow SH *et al.* (2005) WHO-EORTC classification for cutaneous lymphomas. *Blood*, 105, 3768–3785.

103 Goodlad JR (2019) Cutaneous lymphoma and important differential diagnoses: emphasis on cases with a cytotoxic phenotype. *Diagn Histopathol*, 25, 240–248.

104 Morice WG, Kurtin PJ, Leibson PJ, Tefferi A and Hanson CA (2003) Demonstration of aberrant T-cell and natural killer-cell antigen expression in all cases of granular lymphocytic leukaemia. *Br J Haematol*, 120, 1026–1036.

105 Kwong YL, Chan TSY, Tan D, Kim SJ, Poon LM, Mow B *et al.* (2017) PD1 blockade with pembrolizumab is highly effective in relapsed or refractory NK/T-cell lymphoma failing l-asparaginase. *Blood*, 129, 2437–2442.

106 Béné MC, Nebe T, Bettelheim P, Buldini B, Bumbea H, Kern W *et al.* (2011) Immunophenotyping of acute leukemia and lymphoproliferative disorders: a consensus proposal of the European LeukemiaNet Work Package 10. *Leukemia*, 25, 567–574.

107 Gaipa G, Basso G, Biondi A and Campana D (2013) Detection of minimal residual disease in pediatric acute lymphoblastic leukemia. *Cytometry B Clin Cytom*, 84, 359–369.

108 Theunissen P, Mejstrikova E, Sedek L, van der Sluijs-Gelling AJ, Gaipa G, Bartels M *et al.*; EuroFlow Consortium (2017) Standardized flow cytometry for highly sensitive MRD measurements in B-cell acute lymphoblastic leukemia. *Blood*, 129, 347–357.

109 Gupta S, Devidas M, Loh ML, Raetz EA, Chen S, Wang C *et al.* (2018) Flow-cytometric vs. morphologic assessment of remission in childhood acute lymphoblastic leukemia: a report from the Children's Oncology Group (COG). *Leukemia*, 32, 1370–1379.

110 Schuurhuis GJ, Heuser M, Freeman S, Béné MC, Buccisano F, Cloos J *et al.* (2018) Minimal/measurable residual disease in AML: a consensus document from the European LeukemiaNet MRD Working Party. *Blood*, 131, 1275–1291.

111 Rawstron AC, Fazi C, Agathangelidis A, Villamor N, Letestu R, Nomdedeu J *et al.* (2016) A complementary role of multiparameter flow cytometry and high-throughput sequencing for minimal residual disease detection in chronic lymphocytic leukemia: an European Research Initiative on CLL study. *Leukemia*, 30, 929–936.

112 Ghia P and Rawstron A (2018) Minimal residual disease analysis in chronic lymphocytic leukemia: A way for achieving more personalized treatments. *Leukemia*, 32, 1307–1316.

113 Durrieu F, Geneviève F, Arnoulet C, Brumpt C, Capiod J-C, Degenne M *et al.* (2011) Normal levels of peripheral CD19$^+$CD5$^+$ CLL-like cells: Toward a defined threshold for CLL follow-up—A GEIL-GOELAMS study. *Cytometry Part B*, 80B, 346–353.

114 Ortiz-Maldonado V, Villamor N, Baumann T, Aymerich M, Magnano L, Mozas P *et al.* (2018) Is there a role for minimal residual disease monitoring in the management of patients with hairy-cell leukaemia? *Br J Haematol*, 183, 127–129.

115 Flores-Montero J, de Tute R, Paiva B, Perez JJ, Bottcher S, Wind H *et al.* (2016) Immunophenotype of normal vs. myeloma plasma cells: Toward antibody panel specifications for MRD detection in multiple myeloma. *Cytometry*, 90B, 61–72.

116 Djokic M, Björklund E, Blennow E, Mazur J, Söderhäll S and Porwit A (2009) Overexpression of CD123 correlates with the hyperdiploid genotype in acute lymphoblastic leukemia. *Haematologica*, 94, 1016–1019.

117 Roshal M, Fromm JR, Winter SS, Dunsmore KP and Wood BL (2010) Immaturity associated antigens are lost during induction for T cell lymphoblastic leukemia: Implications for minimal residual disease detection. *Cytom B Clin Cytom*, 78, 139–145.

118 Illingworth AJ, Marinov I and Sutherland DR (2019) Sensitive and accurate identification of PNH clones based on ICSS/ESCCA PNH Consensus Guidelines. *Int J Lab Haematol*, 41, Suppl. S1, 73–81.

119 Bain BJ, Clark DM and Wilkins BS (2019) *Bone Marrow Pathology, 5th edn.* Wiley-Blackwell, Oxford pp. 645–684.

Bibliography

Bain BJ (2017) *Leukaemia Diagnosis*, 5th edn. Wiley Blackwell, Oxford.

Keren DF, McCoy JP and Carey JL (2007) *Flow Cytometry in Clinical Diagnosis*, 4th edn. ASCP Press, Chicago.

Leach M, Drummond M and Doig A (2013) *Practical Flow Cytometry in Haematology Diagnosis*, Wiley-Blackwell.

Leach M, Drummond M, Doig A, McKay P, Jackson R and Bain BJ (2015) *Practical Flow Cytometry in Haematology: 100 worked examples*. Wiley, Oxford.

Matutes E, Bain BJ and Wotherspoon A (2020) *Lymphoid malignancies*, 2nd edn, Clinical Publishing.

Ortolani C (2011) *Flow Cytometry in Haematological Malignancies*. Wiley-Blackwell, Oxford.

Porwit A and Béné MC (eds) (2018) *Multiparameter Flow Cytometry in the Diagnosis of Hematologic Malignancies*, Cambridge University Press, Cambridge.

Swerdlow SH, Campo E, Harris NL, Jaffe ES, Pileri S, Stein H and Thiele J (eds) (2017) *WHO Classification of Tumours of Haematopoietic and Lymphoid Tissues*, revised 4th edn. IARC Press, Lyon.

Websites

http://www.pathologyoutlines.com/

https://www.nordiqc.org/epitope.php?id=55 NordiQC Immunohistochemistry Quality Control.

http://www.haematologyetc.co.uk/Marker_description Manchester Haematological Cancers Diagnostic Partnership

https://www.flowcytometrynet.com

Part 4

Test Yourself

CONTENTS

This chapter comprises multiple-choice questions, both Short Answer Questions (SAQs) and Extended Matching Questions (EMQs) so that readers can test their knowledge of immunophenotyping. In addition, there are questions based on case studies that integrate flow cytometry with other clinicopathological data. The first three sections of this book should provide enough information to permit interpretation of the immunophenotype but knowledge of other clinicopathological features is also tested. For this reason, we anticipate that the questions will be particularly useful for those undertaking Royal College of Pathologists examinations (although some of them are more difficult than would be expected in this examination). Magnification of images is shown as the objective used in photography.

Abbreviations

κ, kappa light chain; λ, lambda light chain; ALL, acute lymphoblastic leukaemia; AML, acute myeloid leukaemia; AST, aspartate transaminase; ATLL, adult T-cell leukaemia/lymphoma; c, cytoplasmic; CD, cluster of differentiation; CML, chronic myeloid leukaemia; CSF, cerebrospinal fluid; CT, computed tomography; EBV, Epstein–Barr virus; EMQ, extended matching question; FBC, full blood count; FISH, fluorescence *in situ* hybridisation; FSC, forward scatter of light; Hb, haemoglobin concentration; HHV, human herpesvirus; HIV, human immunodeficiency virus; HTLV-1, human T-cell lymphotropic virus 1; ITD, internal tandem duplication; LDH, lactate dehydrogenase; LGL, large granular lymphocyte; MDS, myelodysplastic syndrome; MPAL, mixed phenotype acute leukaemia; MPO, myeloperoxidase; MRI, magnetic resonance imaging; NK, natural killer; NR, normal range; SAQ, short answer question; SSC, side scatter of light; Sm, surface membrane; TdT, terminal deoxynucleotidyl transferase; ULN, upper limit of normal; WBC, white blood cell count; WHO, World Health Organization.

Immunophenotyping for Haematologists: Principles and Practice, First Edition. Barbara J. Bain and Mike Leach.
© 2021 John Wiley & Sons Ltd. Published 2021 by John Wiley & Sons Ltd.

Short Answer Questions (Single Best Answer)

SAQ 1

A 48-year-old man presents with symptoms of lethargy and night sweats. He is found to have hepatosplenomegaly and generalised lymphadenopathy. His FBC shows anaemia and lymphocytosis with mild thrombocytopenia. Chest radiography shows small bilateral pleural effusions. A blood film shows predominantly small lymphocytes with a high nucleocytoplasmic ratio and weakly basophilic cytoplasm; some nuclei have deep narrow clefts. Immunophenotyping shows expression of CD10, CD19, CD20, CD79b, FMC7 and Smλ. There is no expression of CD5, CD19, CD23, CD34, CD43, CD200 or TdT.

I) The most likely diagnosis is
 A) B-lineage ALL
 B) Burkitt lymphoma
 C) Follicular lymphoma
 D) Primary effusion lymphoma
 E) Small lymphocytic lymphoma

II) The most likely cytogenetic abnormality is
 1) t(8;14)(q24.2;q32)
 2) t(11;14)(q13;q32)
 3) t(12;21)(p13.2;q22.1)
 4) t(14;18)(q32;q21)
 5) Trisomy 12

SAQ 2

A 72-year-old man presents with symptoms of anaemia. His FBC and film show a WBC of $18.6 \times 10^9/l$ with an increased number of cells resembling large lymphocytes; these constitute 25% of peripheral blood cells and have a high nucleocytoplasmic ratio and moderately basophilic cytoplasm. Immunophenotyping shows expression of CD20, CD38, CD56, CD138 (strong), nuclear cyclin D1 and cytoplasmic λ. There is no expression of CD5, CD19 or CD23.

I) The most likely diagnosis is
 A) Chronic lymphocytic leukaemia
 B) Lymphoplasmacytic lymphoma
 C) Mantle cell lymphoma
 D) Plasma cell leukaemia
 E) Small lymphocytic lymphoma

II) The most likely cytogenetic abnormality is
 1) del(13q)
 2) del(17p)
 3) t(11;14)(q13;q32)
 4) t(14;18)(q23;q21)
 5) Trisomy 12

SAQ 3

A 67-year-old woman presents with fatigue and bruising and is found to have generalised lymphadenopathy. Her FBC shows WBC $73 \times 10^9/l$, Hb 72 g/l and platelet count $15 \times 10^9/l$. Her blood film shows an abnormal population of medium-sized cells with a high nucleocytoplasmic ratio and indistinct nucleoli; no cytoplasmic granules are apparent. Immunophenotyping show expression of CD10, CD13, CD19, CD25, CD33, CD66 and TdT. There is no expression of CD5, CD34, MPO, κ or λ.

I) The most likely diagnosis is
 A) Acute myeloid leukaemia
 B) B-lineage ALL
 C) Burkitt lymphoma
 D) Mixed phenotype acute leukaemia
 E) T-lineage ALL

II) The most likely cytogenetic abnormality is
 1) High hyperdiploidy
 2) t(1;19)(q23;p13.3)
 3) t(4;11)(q21;q23.3)
 4) t(9;22)(q34.1;q11.2)
 5) t(12;21)(p13.2;q22.1)

SAQ 4

A 52-year-old man presents with pneumonia and is found to have splenomegaly. His FBC shows: WBC $30 \times 10^9/l$, Hb 87 g/l, platelets $57 \times 10^9/l$, neutrophils $2.3 \times 10^9/l$, lymphocytes

26×10^9/l, monocytes 0.9×10^9/l and eosinophils 0.6×10^9/l. Some lymphocytes have prominent nucleoli and irregular cytoplasmic margins. Immunophenotyping show an abnormal population of cells expressing CD11c, CD19, CD20, CD45, CD103, FMC7 and strong Smκ. There is no expression of CD25, CD123, CD200 or Smλ.

I) The most likely diagnosis is
   A) Blastic plasmacytoid dendritic cell neoplasm
   B) Hairy cell leukaemia
   C) Hairy cell leukaemia variant
   D) Splenic lymphoma with villous lymphocytes
   E) Splenic marginal zone lymphoma

II) Further investigations would be likely to show
   1) Annexin A1 expression
   2) *BRAF* mutation
   3) *KLFR* mutation
   4) *MYD88* mutation
   5) None of the above

SAQ5

A 40-year-old man presents with fever, sweating and hepatosplenomegaly. His FBC and blood film show anaemia, neutropenia and thrombocytopenia with abnormal circulating cells, which are larger than normal lymphocytes with somewhat irregular nuclei and plentiful cytoplasm containing azurophilic granules. Immunophenotyping shows expression of CD2, CD16 and CD56. There is no expression of SmCD3, CD5 or CD57. On immunohistochemistry of a trephine biopsy section, there is expression of CD2, CD3ε and CD56, and EBV is detected.

I) The most likely diagnosis is
   A) Aggressive NK-cell leukaemia
   B) Chronic lymphoproliferative disorder of NK cells
   C) Extranodal NK/T-cell lymphoma, nasal type

D) Infectious mononucleosis
E) T-cell large granular lymphocytic leukaemia

II) This condition is most often observed in
   1) Afro-Caribbeans
   2) Arabs
   3) Chinese
   4) Indians/Pakistanis
   5) Northern European Caucasians

SAQ 6

A 32-year-old pregnant woman presents with bilateral breast enlargement and an abdominal mass. She is found to have diffuse infiltration of the bone marrow by medium-sized cells with a high nucleocytoplasmic ratio and strongly basophilic, vacuolated cytoplasm. These cells express CD10 (weakly), CD19, CD20, CD22, CD38 (strongly), CD43 and Smκ. They do not express CD5, CD34, CD138, Smλ or TdT.

I) The most likely diagnosis is
   A) B-ALL
   B) Blastic plasmacytoid dendritic cell neoplasm
   C) Burkitt lymphoma
   D) Diffuse large B-cell lymphoma
   E) Prolymphocytic leukaemia

II) A trephine biopsy section is stained with the Ki-67 monoclonal antibody. The proliferation fraction is likely to be
   1) 5%
   2) 15%
   3) 25%
   4) 50%
   5) 95% or higher

SAQ 7

A 64-year-old woman presents with a 2-week history of worsening abdominal pain, reduced oral intake, lethargy and fever. Her FBC shows WBC 151×10^9/l, Hb 119 g/l and platelet count 33×10^9/l. Her blood film shows numerous blast cells with moderately basophilic cytoplasm, some with a prominent nuclear indentation. Some blast cells are granular, and some contain 1–3 Auer rods. Immunophenotyping shows expression of CD33 (strong), CD117 and CD123 with partial expression of HLA-DR and MPO. There is no expression of CD11b, CD13, CD14, CD34 or CD64.

I) The most likely diagnosis is
  A) Acute promyelocytic leukaemia
  B) AML, not otherwise specified
  C) AML with biallelic mutation of *CEBPA*
  D) AML with mutated *NPM1*
  E) Blastic plasmacytoid dendritic cell neoplasm

II) Mutation is most likely to be found in
  1) *CEBPA*
  2) *NPM1*
  3) *NPM1* and *FLT3*
  4) *PML*
  5) *RARA*

SAQ 8

A 42-year-old Afro-Caribbean man presents with diplopia and is found to have a left 6th nerve palsy and skin infiltration. Examination of cerebrospinal fluid shows increased protein concentration and increased lymphocytes, some with irregular or highly lobulated nuclei but without cytoplasmic granules. Immunophenotyping shows expression of CD2, CD3, CD5, CD4 and CD25. There is no expression of CD7, CD8, CD34 or TdT.

I) The most likely diagnosis is
  A) Adult T-cell leukaemia/lymphoma
  B) ALK-positive anaplastic large cell lymphoma
  C) Sézary syndrome
  D) T-ALL
  E) T-prolymphocytic leukaemia

II) The virus most likely to be implicated in the pathogenesis is
  1) Epstein–Barr virus
  2) Human herpesvirus 7
  3) Human herpesvirus 8
  4) Human immunodeficiency virus
  5) Human T-cell lymphotropic virus 1

SAQ 9

A 23-year-old man presents with fatigue and pruritus and is found to have splenomegaly. His FBC shows WBC 25×10^9/l, Hb 119 g/l, platelet count 333×10^9/l, neutrophil count 8.4×10^9/l and eosinophil count 15.3×10^9/l. His blood film shows that some eosinophils are hypogranular, some are vacuolated and some have non-lobated nuclei. There is no monocytosis and no blast cells or granulocyte precursors are seen. Bone marrow aspiration and trephine biopsy show a hypercellular marrow with increased eosinophils and precursors; in addition, the trephine biopsy sections show abnormal cells that are thought to be mast cells, in loose non-cohesive clusters. Cytogenetic analysis is normal. Fluorescence *in situ* hybridization shows deletion of the *CHIC2* gene.

I) The most likely diagnosis is
  A) Atypical chronic myeloid leukaemia
  B) Chronic myeloid leukaemia
  C) Myeloproliferative neoplasm with *PDGFRA* rearrangement
  D) Reactive eosinophilia
  E) Systemic mastocytosis

II) The most reliable immunohistochemical marker to confirm the suspicion of increased mast cells is
  1) CD68
  2) CD117
  3) Co-expression of CD2 and CD25
  4) Mast cell chymotryptase
  5) Mast cell tryptase

Extended Matching Questions

EMQ 1

A) Acute megakaryoblastic leukaemia with t(1;22)(p13.3;q13.1)
B) Acute promyelocytic leukaemia with t(15;17)(q24.1;q21.2)
C) AML with inv(16)(p13.1q22)
D) AML with *NPM1* mutation
E) AML with t(6;9)(p23;q34.1)
F) AML with t(8;21)(q22;q22.1)
G) AML with t(9;11)(p21.3;q23.3)
H) Early T-cell precursor acute lymphoblastic leukaemia
I) Mixed phenotype acute leukaemia
J) T-ALL

For each clinicopathological description below, select the most likely diagnosis from the list of options above. Each option may be used once, more than once, or not at all.

1) A 23-year-old woman presents with epistaxis and bruising. Her FBC shows WBC 21.0×10^9/l, Hb 110 g/l and platelet count 25×10^9/l. There are medium-sized cells with bilobed nuclei; some have fine cytoplasmic granules. Her bone marrow is largely replaced by similar cells. Immunophenotyping shows these to express CD13 (heterogeneous), CD33 (strong), CD117 (weak) and MPO (strong). There is no expression of CD34 or HLA-DR.

2) A 2-year-old child appears pale, lethargic and irritable. He is found to have marked hepatosplenomegaly. His FBC shows WBC 25×10^9/l, Hb 76 g/l and platelet count 56×10^9/l. There are abnormal, medium-sized blast cells with a high nucleocytoplasmic ratio, basophilic blebbed cytoplasm and no apparent granules. Immunophenotyping shows these to express CD13, CD33, CD41 and CD61. CD34 and MPO are not expressed.

3) A 42-year-old man presents with tiredness and low-grade fever. His spleen is just palpable and he has some bruises. His FBC shows WBC 62×10^9/l, Hb 102 g/l and platelet count 78×10^9/l. 90% of circulating cells are blast cells of variable appearance, ranging from small cells with scanty cytoplasm to medium-sized cells with more abundant, weakly basophilic, agranular cytoplasm. Immunophenotyping shows expression of MPO, cCD3 but not SmCD3, CD9 (weak), CD19 (strong), CD79a and cCD22 but not SmCD22. FISH shows rearrangement of *KMT2A*.

4) A 23-year-old woman presents with general malaise. Her FBC shows WBC 22×10^9/l, Hb 92 g/l and platelet count 82×10^9/l. 65% of circulating cells are granular blast cells, some with a single long Auer rod. There is also mild eosinophilia and mature neutrophils appear dysplastic. Immunophenotyping of the blast cells shows expression of CD13, CD19, CD33, CD34, CD56, CD65, CD79a, CD117, HLA-DR and MPO. FISH shows *RUNX1-RUNX1T1* fusion.

5) A 10-year-old boy presents with lymphadenopathy and splenomegaly. His FBC show leucocytosis, anaemia and thrombocytopenia. His blood film shows small to medium-sized blast cells with a high nucleocytoplasmic ratio and no apparent granules. Immunophenotyping shows expression of cCD3, CD7, CD11b, CD13, CD33, CD65 and CD117. There is no expression of CD1a, CD4, CD8, or MPO.

EMQ 2

A) Chronic lymphocytic leukaemia
B) Follicular lymphoma
C) Hairy cell leukaemia
D) Hairy cell leukaemia variant
E) Lymphoplasmacytic lymphoma
F) Mantle cell lymphoma
G) Mucosa-associated lymphoid tissue (MALT) lymphoma
H) Persistent polyclonal B-cell lymphocytosis
I) Prolymphocytic leukaemia
J) Splenic marginal zone lymphoma

For each clinicopathological description below, select the most likely diagnosis from the list of options above. Each option may be used once, more than once, or not at all.

1) A 65-year-old woman presents with malaise and fatigue. She is found to have splenomegaly and generalised lymphadenopathy. Her FBC shows anaemia and lymphocytosis and a blood film shows abnormal, medium-sized lymphocytes, some with irregular or cleft nuclei and some with nucleoli. Immunophenotyping shows a population of cells expressing CD5, CD19, CD20, CD43, CD45, CD79b, FMC7 and moderate λ. There is no expression of CD2, CD3, CD10, CD23, CD200 or κ. On histological sections, there is expression of cyclin D1, BCL2 and SOX11 but not of BCL6.

2) A 67-year-old man is being followed in outpatients because of chronic kidney disease and hypertension. Apart from reduced pulses in his legs, there are no abnormal physical findings. A routine FBC shows WBC $45 \times 10^9/l$, Hb 132 g/l, lymphocyte count $37 \times 10^9/l$ and platelet count $135 \times 10^9/l$. Immunophenotyping shows expression of CD5, CD19, CD20 (weak), CD22 (weak), CD23, CD38, CD43, CD45, CD79b (weak), CD200 and Smκ (weak). There is no expression of FMC7 or Smλ.

3) A 32-year-old woman is found to have lymphocytosis (lymphocyte count $5.4 \times 10^9/l$) with no abnormal physical findings. She smokes 20 cigarettes a day and on average drinks 1–2 units of alcohol per day. Her blood film shows binucleated lymphocytes and immunophenotyping shows expression of CD19, CD20, CD24, CD25, CD79b and FMC7. Some cells express κ light chain and some λ.

4) A 64-year-old man presents with recurrent infections and is found to have moderate splenomegaly. FBC shows pancytopenia, including monocytopenia. There are infrequent abnormal cells in the peripheral blood. These show expression of CD11c, CD19, CD20 (strong), CD22 (strong), CD25, CD45, CD103, CD123 and CD200 (strong).

5) A 52-year-old man presents with splenomegaly and anaemia. His spleen is palpable 10 cm below the left costal margin. There is no lymphadenopathy. His FBC shows WBC $14 \times 10^9/l$, Hb 102 g/l, lymphocyte count $6.5 \times 10^9/l$ and platelet count $130 \times 10^9/l$. The lymphocytes are mainly small with a round nucleus, no apparent nucleolus and a moderate amount of weakly basophilic cytoplasm. Some have irregular cytoplasmic margins, sometimes with polar villi. A minority have more basophilic cytoplasm and a paranuclear Golgi zone. Immunophenotyping shows expression of CD19, CD20, CD79b, FMC7 and Smκ. There is no expression of CD5, CD10, CD11c, CD23, CD25, CD43, CD45, CD103 or CD123.

EMQ 3

A) Adult T-cell leukaemia/lymphoma (ATLL)
B) Aggressive NK-cell leukaemia
C) Angioimmunoblastic T-cell lymphoma (AITCL)
D) Blastic plasmacytoid dendritic cell neoplasm (BPDCN)
E) Chronic lymphoproliferative disorder of NK cells
F) Mycosis fungoides (MF)
G) Sézary syndrome (SS)
H) T-cell large granular lymphocytic leukaemia (T-LGLL)
I) T-cell prolymphocytic leukaemia (T-PLL)
J) T lymphoblastic leukaemia/lymphoma (T-ALL)

For each clinicopathological description below, select the most likely diagnosis from the list of options above. Each option may be used once, more than once, or not at all.

1) A 65-year-old man presents with hepatosplenomegaly. He is found to have lymphocytosis (lymphocyte count $36 \times 10^9/l$). His blood film shows medium-sized lymphoid cells with irregular nuclei showing dense chromatin and the presence of a medium-sized nucleolus; there is scanty basophilic cytoplasmic with some cytoplasmic blebs. Immunophenotyping shows expression of CD2, CD3, CD4, CD5, CD7, CD8 and weak CD25. CD1a and TdT are negative.

2) A 60-year-old woman presents with lymphadenopathy. She is found to be anaemic with increased medium-sized lymphoid cells in the peripheral blood; these have a diffuse chromatin pattern and ill-defined nucleoli. Immunophenotyping shows expression of cCD3, CD1a, CD4, CD7, CD8 and TdT. There is no expression of CD4 or SmCD3.

3) A 70-year-old man presents with hepatosplenomegaly and skin infiltration. He has recently suffered from *Pneumocystis jirovecii* pneumonia. He is found to be hypercalcaemic and has lymphocytosis. His blood film shows medium-size, pleomorphic cells, some with lobulated nuclei. Immunophenotyping shows expression of CD2, CD3 (weak), CD4, CD5, CD25, CD38 and HLA-DR.

4) A 70-year-old man presents with recurrent infection and is found to have neutropenia and lymphocytosis. He is known to suffer from rheumatoid arthritis. On physical examination, there are signs of a chest infection. A blood film shows an increase of large granular lymphocytes without any atypical cytological feature. Immunophenotyping shows expression of CD2, CD3, CD8, CD16 and CD57. CD56 is not expressed.

5) A 53-year old man presents with pruritus and a rash. He is found to have lymphadenopathy and lymphocytosis (lymphocyte count $6.2 \times 10^9/l$). His blood film shows a population of small lymphocytes with scanty cytoplasm and irregular and convoluted nuclei. Immunophenotyping shows high side scatter (SSC) and expression of CD2, CD3, CD4 and CD5. There is no expression of CD7 or CD8.

EMQ 4

A) Acute panmyelosis with myelofibrosis
B) Acute undifferentiated leukaemia
C) Anaplastic large cell lymphoma
D) Classical Hodgkin lymphoma
E) Metastatic carcinoma
F) Neuroblastoma
G) Nodular lymphocyte predominant Hodgkin lymphoma
H) Primary mediastinal B-cell lymphoma
I) Primary myelofibrosis
J) Systemic mastocytosis

For each clinicopathological description below, select the most likely diagnosis from the list of options above.

1) A 54-year-old man presents following a sudden collapse. He is found to have a WBC of $4.0 \times 10^9/l$, an Hb of 80 g/l and a platelet count of $45 \times 10^9/l$. A trephine biopsy section is hypercellular and shows swathes of spindle shaped cells, which express CD2, CD25 and CD117.

2) A 57-year-old woman presents with bone pain and fatigue. Her blood count shows WBC $4.2 \times 10^9/l$, Hb 87 g/l and platelet count $482 \times 10^9/l$. Her blood film is leucoerythroblastic with teardrop poikilocytes. Bone marrow cannot be aspirated. Trephine biopsy sections shows myelofibrosis and osteosclerosis. Immunohistochemistry shows a population of cells within the

fibrotic marrow expressing epithelial membrane antigen and oestrogen receptor.

3) A 54-year-old man presents with lymphadenopathy. Biopsy of a lymph node shows an abnormal diffuse infiltrate with large cells expressing CD2, CD4, CD30 and epithelial membrane antigen. CD3 and ALK (CD246) are not expressed.

4) A 34-year-old woman presents with cervical and inguinal lymphadenopathy and a mediastinal mass. Lymph node and trephine biopsies are performed. The latter shows focal infiltration by large mononuclear cells with prominent nucleoli on a background of small lymphocytes and eosinophils. No Reed–Sternberg cells are seen. The large cells express CD15, CD30, weak PAX5 and weak CD20 in a proportion of cells.

5) A 70-year-old man presents with fatigue, weakness and bone pain. On examination, the only abnormality detected is pallor. His FBC shows pancytopenia and borderline macrocytosis. Bone marrow cannot be aspirated. Trephine biopsy sections show increased immature cells in a fibrotic background. CD34 is expressed by more than 20% of cells. There are also populations of cells expressing, respectively, CD117, E-cadherin and CD42b.

FRCPath-Type Questions

The questions that follow are similar to those used in the final examination for the fellowship of the Royal College or Pathologists (FRCPath). For advanced trainees in haematology to gain maximum benefit from these, it is important to work out your answers before looking at the authors' preferred answers.

Case 1

The FBC of a newborn baby girl shows WBC 27.8×10^9/l, Hb 188 g/l, MCV 119 fl and platelet count 200×10^9/l. The differential count shows neutrophils 16.1×10^9/l, blast cells 10.3×10^9/l and nucleated red blood cells 2.1×10^9/l.

A representative blood film image is shown in Figure 4.1.

Immunophenotyping of the abnormal cells shows CD34+, CD117−, CD13−, CD33+, HLA-DR+, CD7+, CD11b+, CD41+, CD61+, CD42b+, cCD3−, CD79a− and MPO−. Other B- and T- lineage markers are negative.

1) Discuss the most likely diagnosis, giving your reasons.
2) What is the question you would ask the clinical staff?

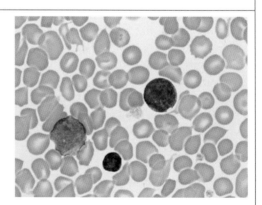

Figure 4.1 (×100)

3) What further tests and other immunophenotypic markers might have been informative?

Case 2

A 72-year-old man on ponatinib therapy for refractory chronic myeloid leukaemia (CML) presents with recurrent pleural effusions. Computed tomography (CT) imaging also showed mediastinal and hilar lymphadenopathy. His FBC shows Hb 123 g/l, WBC 6 × 10^9/l, neutrophils 4.2 × 10^9/l and platelets 115 × 10^9/l.

Pleural fluid is aspirated. The WBC is 0.91 × 10^9/l (upper limit of normal (ULN) 0.001 × 10^9/l).

Cytospin preparations are shown in Figures 4.2a and b.

Gating on CD34+ events is done and shows CD117+, CD13−, CD33−, HLA-DR−, CD7+, CD56+, CD10+, cCD3+, SmCD3−, CD2−, CD5−, CD4−, CD8−, TdT−, CD79a−, CD19− and MPO−.

Cytogenetic analysis shows 48,XY,+X, t(9;22)(q34.1;q11.2),+ider(22)(q10)

1) What do the morphology and flow cytometry findings indicate?
2) Is this an expected event?

(a)

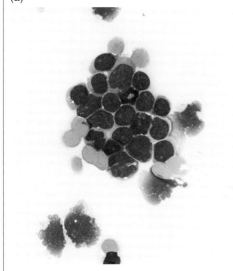

Figure 4.2a   (×50)

(b)

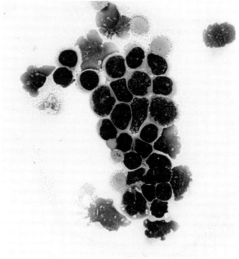

Figure 4.2b   (×50)

Case 3

A 57-year-old man previously treated with allogeneic transplantation for acute myeloid leukaemia presents with headache and altered sensation over his face. His FBC shows Hb 117 g/l, WBC 2.4 × 10^9/l, neutrophils 1.1 × 10^9/l and platelets 45 × 10^9/l.

Magnetic resonance imaging (MRI) of the brain shows no abnormality. CSF is obtained, showing WBC 1.29 × 10^9/l and protein 5.98 g/l (ULN 0.5).

A CSF cytospin preparation is shown in Figures 4.3a and b.

1) What is the most likely diagnosis?

(a)

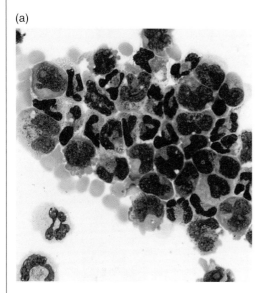

Figure 4.3a   (×50)

(b)

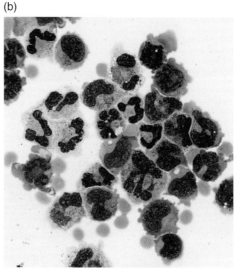

Figure 4.3b   (×50)

Case 4

An 83-year-old woman presented with progressive weight loss. Her FBC shows Hb 103 g/l, WBC 6.8 × 10⁹/l, neutrophils 4.3 × 10⁹/l and platelets 62 × 10⁹/l. Her blood film is leucoerythroblastic. Serum lactate dehydrogenase (LDH) is 1400 iu/l (ULN 250).

CT imaging showed extensive mediastinal and para-aortic lymphadenopathy and lymphoma is suspected.

A bone marrow aspirate is taken and is shown in Figures 4.4a and b.

The large non-granular cells were gated for analysis (CD45 negative cells on CD45/SSC) (Figure 4.4c). Flow cytometry shows CD34−, CD117+, CD13−, CD33−, HLA-DR+, CD56+, cCD3−, CD79a− and MPO−. Other T- and B-lineage markers are negative.

1) What is the most likely diagnosis?

(a)

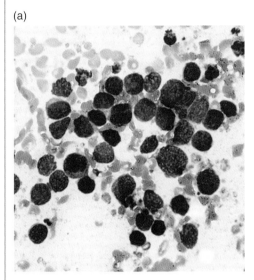

Figure 4.4a (×50)

(b)

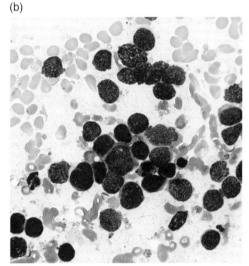

Figure 4.4b (×50)

(c)

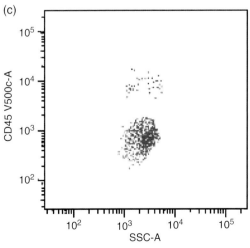

Figure 4.4c

Case 5

A 50-year-old man presents with fatigue and pallor. His FBC shows Hb 79 g/l, WBC 43.9 × 10^9/l and platelets 49 × 10^9/l.

His blood film is shown in Figures 4.5a and b.

Immunophenotyping is performed with gating on large cells (Figures 4.5c and d).

1) What is the most likely diagnosis?
2) Explain whether this is confirmed by the immunophenotype shown.

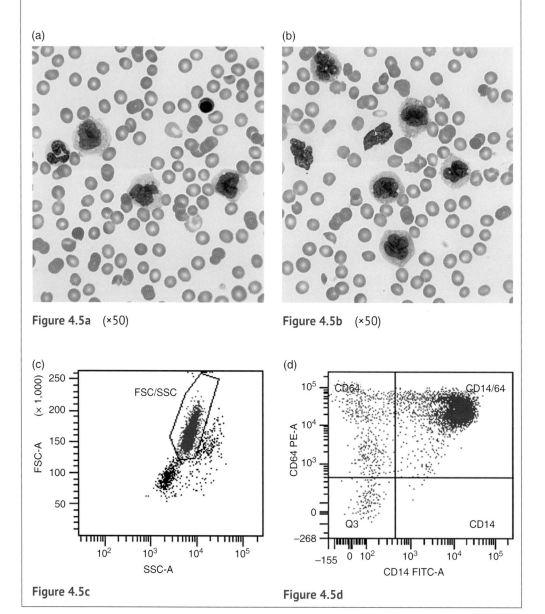

(a)

Figure 4.5a (×50)

(b)

Figure 4.5b (×50)

(c)

Figure 4.5c

(d)

Figure 4.5d

Case 6

A 70-year-old man presents with purplish nodular skin infiltrates. His FBC shows Hb 115 g/l, WBC 50 × 10⁹/l and platelets 27 × 10⁹/l.

His blood film is shown in Figures 4.6a and b.

The large blastoid cells are gated for analysis with some data shown in Figures 4.6c–f.

The full immunophenotype is CD33+, HLA-DR+, CD4+, CD7+, CD123+, CD56+, CD34−, CD117−, cCD3−, CD15−, CD64−, CD79a−, CD19− and MPO−.

Cytogenetic analysis shows 46,XY.

1) How do you interpret the immunophenotype?
2) What is your working diagnosis?

(a)

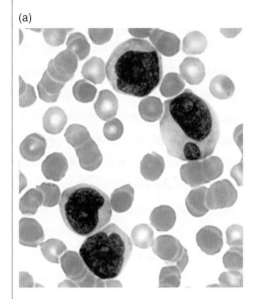

Figure 4.6a   (×100)

(b)

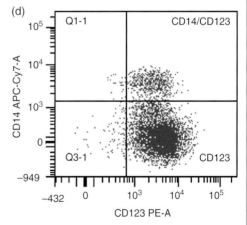

Figure 4.6b   (×100)

(c)

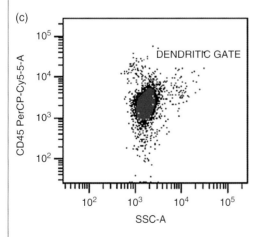

Figure 4.6c

(d)

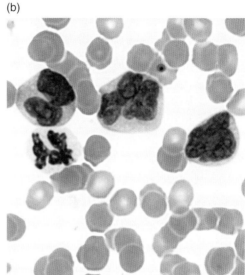

Figure 4.6d

(*continued*)

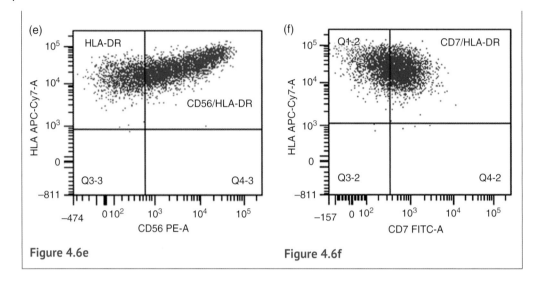

Figure 4.6e

Figure 4.6f

Case 7

A 90-year-old woman, who is known to the haematology clinic, presented with a rapid clinical decline. Her FBC shows Hb 81 g/l, WBC 52 × 10⁹/l and platelets 71 × 10⁹/l.

Her blood film is shown in Figures 4.7a and b.

1) What is your working diagnosis?
2) How do you explain the red cell morphology?
3) What extramedullary tissues can be affected by this disease?

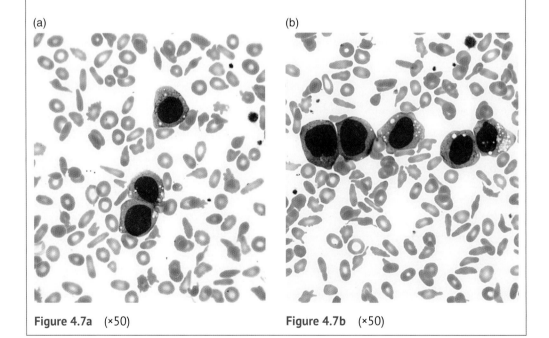

Figure 4.7a   (×50)

Figure 4.7b   (×50)

Case 8

A 45-year-old man presents with fatigue. He had received chemoradiotherapy for a squamous carcinoma of the oropharynx 3 years previously. His blood count shows Hb 111 g/l, WBC 447 × 10⁹/l and platelets 18 × 10⁹/l.

His blood film is shown in Figures 4.8a and b.

1) State the most likely diagnosis, giving your reasons.

Flow cytometry studies gating on CD34+ cells show CD117–, CD15+, HLA-DR+, CD19+, CD10–, CD20–, cCD3–, CD79a+ and MPO–.

2) What is your final diagnosis and what molecular abnormality do you suspect?

(a)

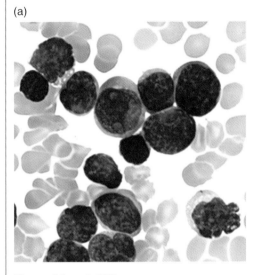

Figure 4.8a   (×100)

(b)

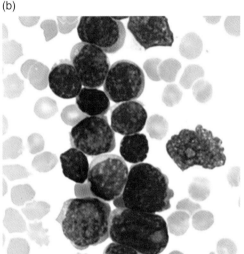

Figure 4.8b   (×100)

Case 9

An 18-year-old man presents with fatigue and pallor. On clinical examination, he has widespread small volume lymphadenopathy. His FBC shows Hb 112 g/l, WBC 34 × 10⁹/l and platelets 33 × 10⁹/l.

His blood film is shown in Figures 4.9a and b and his immunophenotype flow plots are shown in Figures 4.9c–e.

The immunophenotyping data gating on cells showing weak CD45 expression shows cCD3+, CD7+, SmCD3–, CD5–, CD4–, CD8–, CD79a+, CD19–, CD10–, CD34–, CD117–, CD13–, CD33–, MPO–, CD14– and CD64–.

Cytogenetic analysis shows 46,XY.

1) State the diagnosis, giving your reasons.

(continued)

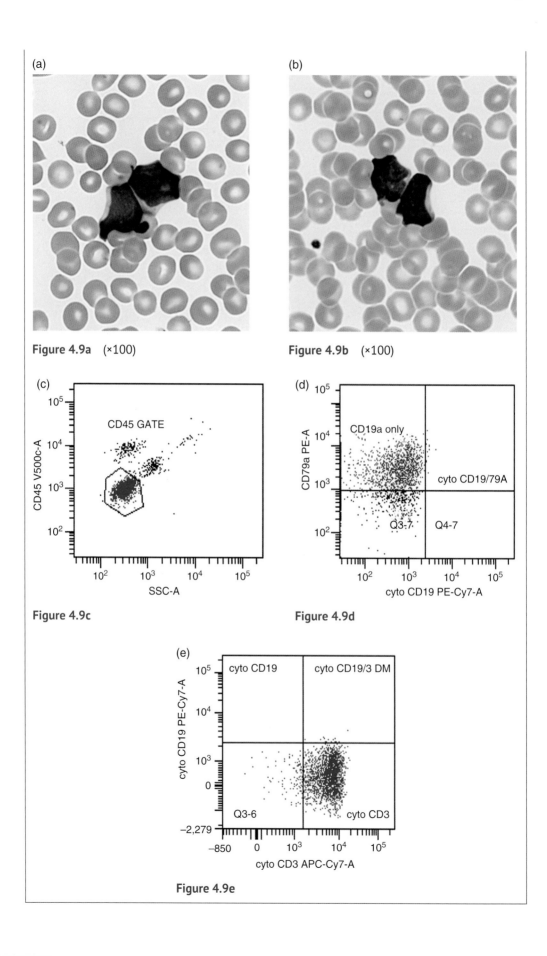

(a)

Figure 4.9a (×100)

(b)

Figure 4.9b (×100)

(c)

CD45 V500c-A

CD45 GATE

10^5
10^4
10^3
10^2

10^2 10^3 10^4 10^5
SSC-A

Figure 4.9c

(d)

CD79a PE-A

CD19a only

cyto CD19/79A

Q3-7 Q4-7

10^5
10^4
10^3
10^2

10^2 10^3 10^4 10^5
cyto CD19 PE-Cy7-A

Figure 4.9d

(e)

cyto CD19 PE-Cy7-A

cyto CD19 cyto CD19/3 DM

Q3-6 cyto CD3

10^5
10^4
10^3
0
−2,279

−850 0 10^3 10^4 10^5
cyto CD3 APC-Cy7-A

Figure 4.9e

Case 10

A 46-year-old man presents with a short history of fatigue and night sweats. His FBC shows Hb 127 g/l, WBC 62 × 10⁹/l, neutrophils 40 × 10⁹/l, eosinophils 0.3 × 10⁹/l, lymphocytes 12 × 10⁹/l and platelets 76 × 10⁹/l.

His blood film is shown in Figures 4.10a and b.

Immunophenotyping studies with gating on the small lymphoid cells (Figure 4.10c) shows CD2−, cCD3+, CD7+, CD5−, CD4−, CD8−, CD26+, HLA-DR+, CD79a−, CD19−, CD10− and CD30+.

Cytogenetic analysis shows 47,XY,ins(2)(2,5)(p23;q35q13),+7.

1) What diagnosis would you suspect from the blood film?
2) Integrating the clinical, morphological, immunophenotypic and cytogenetic data, what is your final diagnosis?

(a)

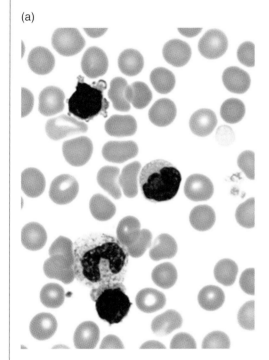

Figure 4.10a   (×100)

(b)

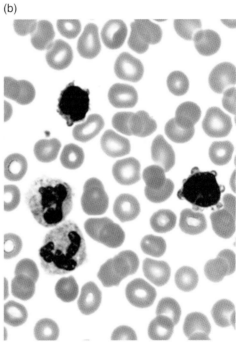

Figure 4.10b   (×100)

(c)

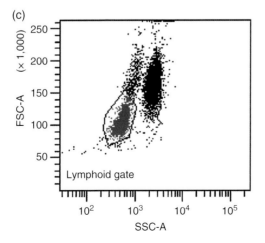

Figure 4.10c

Case 11

A 15-year-old male presents with jaundice and pallor following an episode of diarrhoea and vomiting. His FBC shows Hb 104 g/l, WBC 12.6 × 10^9/l, neutrophils 8.6 × 10^9/l and platelets 225 × 10^9/l. The reticulocyte count is 287 × 10^9/l (normal range (NR) 50–100). A direct Coombs test is negative. Biochemical tests show serum LDH 370 iu/l (ULN 240) and bilirubin 97 µmol/l with normal transaminases.

His blood film is shown in Figure 4.11.

1) What is your diagnosis?
2) How would you confirm it?

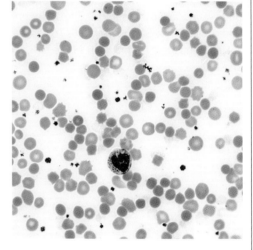

Figure 4.11   (×50)

Case 12

A 48-year-old man is admitted to the urology ward and is reported to have abdominal pain and haematuria. His FBC shows Hb 85 g/l, WBC 6.6 × 10^9/l, neutrophils 5.1 × 10^9/l and platelets 49 × 10^9/l. His reticulocyte count is 113 × 10^9/l (NR 50–100). Biochemical tests show creatinine 81 µmol/l, LDH 711 iu/l (ULN 240), bilirubin 23 µmol/l, aspartate transaminase (AST) 64 (NR<40 u/l), alanine transaminase (ALT) 13 (NR <50 u/l) and alkaline phosphatase 95 (NR 30-130 u/l). Haematinic assays are normal.

His blood film is shown in Figure 4.12.

1) What diagnoses should be considered and why?
2) What specific tests could be useful?

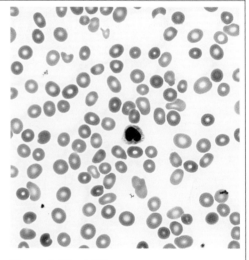

Figure 4.12   (×50)

Case 13

A 73-year-old woman is referred for investigation of lymphocytosis noted at a surgical pre-assessment clinic. No pathological lymph nodes are evident on clinical examination but her spleen tip is palpable. Her FBC shows Hb 145 g/l, WBC 17×10^9/l, neutrophils 2.5×10^9/l, lymphocytes 13.8×10^9/l and platelets 120×10^9/l.

Her blood film is shown in Figures 4.13a and b.

Immunophenotyping studies, gating on CD19+ cells (Figures 4.13c and d), show CD20++, CD22+, CD79b+, CD23–, FMC7+, CD10–, CD200–, kappa++, lambda–, CD3–, CD5+, CD7–, CD4– and CD8–.

Immunohistochemistry on a fixed pellet of peripheral blood lymphocytes shows CD20+, CD5+, cyclin D1–, SOX11– and LEF1–.

1) What is the CLL score?
2) What is the likely diagnosis?
3) What treatment is indicated

(a)

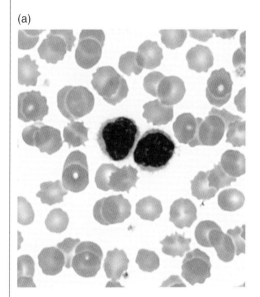

Figure 4.13a   (×100)

(b)

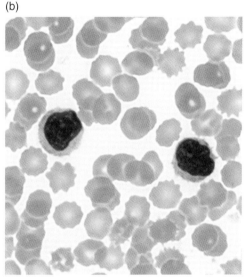

Figure 4.13b   (×100)

(c)

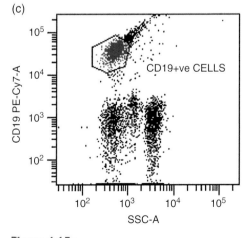

Figure 4.13c

(d)

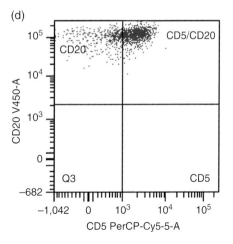

Figure 4.13d

Case 14

A 60-year-old woman presents with pain in the anterior chest and ribs together with a short history of fatigue. A CT pulmonary angiogram shows mediastinal lymphadenopathy. Her blood film shows a small number of circulating blast cells. Her FBC shows Hb 107 g/l, WBC 4.1 × 10⁹/l, neutrophils 1.5 × 10⁹/l, lymphocytes 1.9 × 10⁹/l and platelets 140 × 10⁹/l.

Her bone marrow aspirate is shown in Figures 4.14a and b (×100).

Immunophenotyping on cells showing weak expression of CD45 (Figure 4.14c) shows CD34+, CD117–, CD13+, CD33+, HLA-DR+, CD14–, CD64–, CD7+, CD3–, CD5–, CD2–, CD4–, CD8–, cCD3–, CD79a–, MPO–, CD19–, CD10–, CD20– and TdT+.

Cytogenetic and molecular genetic analysis show 46,XX with no *BCR-ABL1* fusion transcript and no *FLT3* internal tandem duplication (ITD) or *NPM1* mutation.

1) Which two diagnoses should be considered?
2) What would be the diagnosis according to the 2016 WHO classification?

(a)

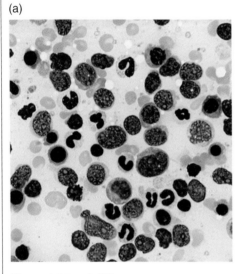

Figure 4.14a (×50)

(b)

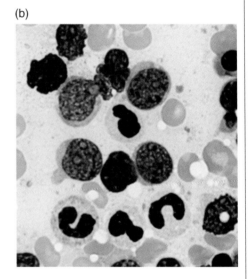

Figure 4.14b (×100)

(c)

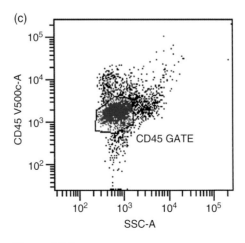

Figure 4.14c

Case 15

A 65-year-old woman is referred for investigation of anaemia and neutropenia. Her FBC shows Hb 84 g/l, WBC 6.1 × 10⁹/l, neutrophils 0.4 × 10⁹/l, lymphocytes 5.1 × 10⁹/l and platelets 105 × 10⁹/l. Her blood film is shown in Figures 4.15a and b.

Gating on lymphoid cells (86% T cells, 2.6% B cells) shows a dominant population with the immunophenotype CD2+, CD3+, CD5–, CD7–, CD4–, CD8+, CD56–, CD57+, CD26– and HLA-DR–. Metaphase cytogenetic analysis is normal.

1) What is the working diagnosis?
2) What further confirmatory investigations are indicated and why are these important?

(a)

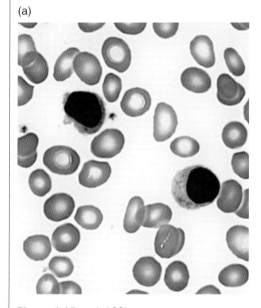

Figure 4.15a   (×100)

(b)

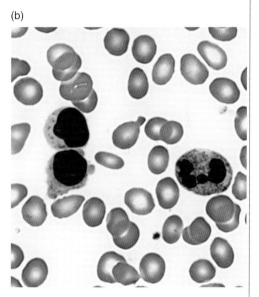

Figure 4.15b   (×100)

Case 16

A 2-year-old girl was referred for investigation of a febrile pneumonic illness associated with anaemia, neutropenia and thrombocytosis. Her FBC showed Hb 95 g/l, WBC 4 × 10⁹/l, neutrophils 1.3 × 10⁹/l and platelets 550 × 10⁹/l. Her blood film was not informative. Her bone marrow aspirate is shown in Figures 4.16a and b. Erythroid, myeloid and megakaryocyte activity was preserved but lymphoid cells were prominent.

Flow cytometric immunophenotyping, gating on CD45^weak cells (15% of events) gave a population with the following phenotype:

CD19+, CD20+, CD79a+, CD10+, TdT + and CD34 +

CD33–, CD13–, CD11b–, MPO–, cCD3–, CD7 – and CD56 –.

Scatter plots are shown in Figures 4.16c –f.
Metaphase cytogenetic analysis was normal.

1) What is your assessment of the bone marrow aspirate?
2) What important features lead you to this conclusion?

(continued)

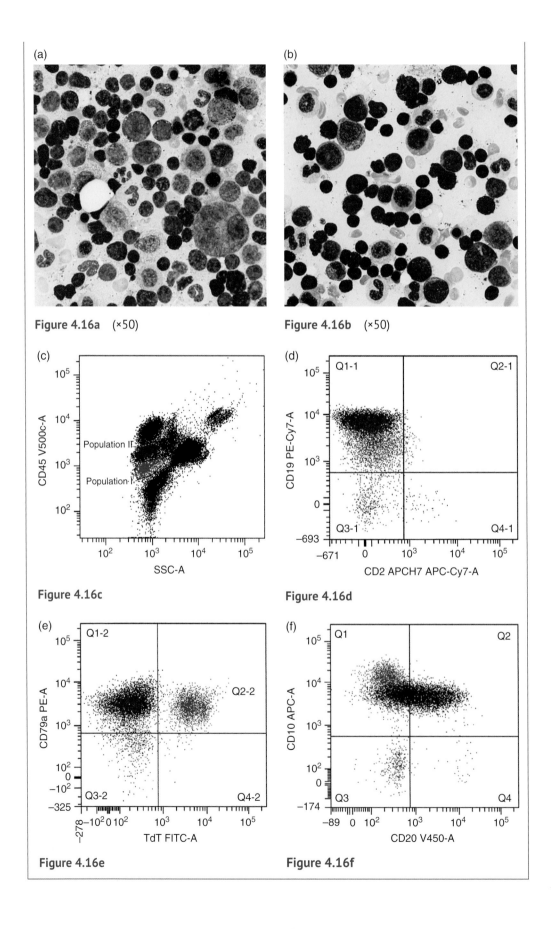

(a)

Figure 4.16a (×50)

(b)

Figure 4.16b (×50)

(c)

Figure 4.16c

(d)

Figure 4.16d

(e)

Figure 4.16e

(f)

Figure 4.16f

Answers to SAQs

SAQ 1

Correct answers: C, 4

This is follicular lymphoma. CD10 expression by circulating lymphoma cells is not always seen but, when positive, can be a pointer to the diagnosis. CD10 would also be expressed in Burkitt lymphoma, but the cytology described would not be typical, and in B-ALL, but the phenotype here is of mature rather than immature B cells. The cytogenetic abnormality expected is t(14;18)(q32;q21) leading to dysregulation of *BCL2* by proximity to the *IGH* locus.

SAQ 2

Correct answers: D, 3

This is plasma cell leukaemia. There is no clue in the described cytological features, which are very variable in this condition, but the immunophenotype reveals the diagnosis and, with 25% circulating neoplastic cells, the criteria of the 2016 revision of the *WHO Classification of Tumours of Haemopoietic and Lymphoid Tissues* [1] are met. The strong expression of CD138 together with CD38 identifies the cells as plasma cells. CD56 is usually positive in multiple myeloma but is positive in only about 20% of cases of plasma cell leukaemia. The expression of cyclin D1 in this case suggests that there is a translocation leading to dysregulation of the *CCND1* gene by proximity to the *IGH* locus, which occurs with t(11;14)(q13;q32) in myeloma and plasma cell leukaemia, as well as in mantle cell lymphoma.

SAQ 3

Correct answers: B, 4

This is B-ALL. Expression of CD13 and CD33 is not sufficient to indicate mixed phenotype acute leukaemia when MPO is negative. The expression of CD13, CD33 and CD66 together with the patient's age make t(9;22) the most likely cytogenetic abnormality. Cases with

t(4;11) can show expression of CD15, whereas the other three genetic categories do not usually show expression of myeloid antigens.

SAQ 4

Correct answers: C, 5

This is hairy cell leukaemia variant. In addition to the lack of expression on CD25 and CD123, the absence of monocytopenia indicates that this is not likely to be hairy cell leukaemia. Annexin A1 expression and *BRAF* mutation are characteristic of hairy cell leukaemia, *KLF2* mutation of splenic marginal zone lymphoma and *MYD88* mutation of lymphoplasmacytic lymphoma. None of these abnormalities is expected in this patient.

SAQ 5

Correct answers: A, 3

This is aggressive NK-cell leukaemia. The expression of CD3ε is a feature of NK cells and is not indicative of a T-cell origin. The clinical picture favours this diagnosis rather than chronic lymphoproliferative disorder of NK cells. The clinical picture and the CD16 expression favour this diagnosis over extranodal NK/T cell lymphoma.

This condition is more common in Chinese.

SAQ 6

Correct answers: C, 5

This is Burkitt lymphoma. Presentation with breast enlargement is associated with puberty, pregnancy and lactation. The proliferation fraction (Ki-67) approaches 100%.

SAQ 7

Correct answers: D, 3

This is AML with mutated *NPM1*. This is suggested by the nuclear invagination and the immunophenotyping is consistent. Some cases have monocytic or myelomonocytic differentiation but others, including this patient, do not. The immunophenotype typically shows expression of CD33 (strong), CD117 and CD123 with HLA-DR often being negative and CD34 usually being negative. Nuclear invagination is associated particularly with the coexistence of an *NPM1* mutation and a *FLT3* internal tandem duplication [2].

Negativity for CD34 and HLA-DR is also characteristic of acute promyelocytic leukaemia, particularly the hypergranular variant, but the description of the morphology is not suggestive of this diagnosis. Acute monoblastic leukaemia is also likely to be CD34-negative, but HLA-DR is typically positive and the description of the cytology does not fit this diagnosis.

SAQ 8

Correct answers: A, 5
This is adult T-cell leukaemia/lymphoma, which occurs only in individuals who are carrying HTLV-1. The virus is clonally integrated in the neoplastic cells. Expression of CD25 is usual. EBV and HIV are implicated in the pathogenesis of many types of lymphoma but not ATLL. HHV8 is implicated in the pathogenesis of primary effusion lymphoma.

SAQ 9

Correct answers: C, 5
The deletion of *CHIC2* in a cytogenetically normal sample shows that there is a cryptic deletion at 4q12. This is indicative of a *FIP1L1-PDGFRA* fusion gene and confirms the diagnosis of myeloproliferative neoplasm with *PDGFRA* rearrangement. There may be increased mast cells in this condition but the diagnosis is not systemic mastocytosis. Mast cell tryptase is more sensitive than mast cell chymotryptase for detection of cells of this lineage, and is more specific than CD117. Neoplastic mast cells often co-express CD2 and CD25 but this is not a lineage marker.

Answers to EMQs

EMQ 1

Correct answers B, A, I, F, H
1) This is the hypogranular/microgranular variant of acute promyelocytic leukaemia. Lack of expression of CD34 and HLA-DR is common (even more so in the hypergranular variant).
2) This is acute megakaryoblastic leukaemia with t(1;22)(p13.3;q13.1). This condition typically presents in children under the age of 3 years. There is expression of megakaryocyte markers, CD41 and CD61. Although these are blast cells (megakaryoblasts), lack of CD34 expression is common.
3) The criteria for mixed phenotype acute leukaemia are met [1]. Because of the FISH finding, the specific diagnosis, according to the 2016 WHO classification, is mixed phenotype acute leukaemia with t(v;11q23.3)/*KMT2A* rearranged.

4) This is AML with t(8;21)(q22;q22.1). It is common in this genetic subtype for there to be expression of CD19; expression of CD79a is not infrequent. Despite the expression of two B-lineage antigens, this is NOT mixed phenotype acute leukaemia. The demonstration of *RUNX1-RUNX1T1* fusion indicates the presence of t(8;21) and precludes the diagnosis of MPAL.
5) This is early T-cell precursor lymphoblastic leukaemia. There is expression of T-cell and myeloid markers but as MPO is not expressed, the criteria for MPAL are not met. The 2016 WHO classification defines this subtype of acute leukaemia on the basis of expression of cCD3 and CD7 plus expression of one or more of specified myeloid and stem cell markers: CD11b, CD13, CD33, CD34, CD65, CD117 and HLA-DR [1]. CD2 and CD4 may be expressed. There is no expression of CD1a, CD8 or MPO.

EMQ 2

Correct answers F, A, H, C, J

1) This is mantle cell lymphoma. The immunophenotype is typical; λ expression is more common than κ [3].
2) This is chronic lymphocytic leukaemia. The immunophenotype is typical. CD38 is expressed in a subset of cases and correlates with a worse prognosis.
3) This is polyclonal B lymphocytosis. The binucleated lymphocytes and the expression of CD25 and both κ and λ are the clues to the diagnosis. This condition is associated with cigarette smoking.
4) This is hairy cell leukaemia. The clue to the diagnosis is in the monocytopenia and the expression of CD11c, CD25, CD103 and CD123.
5) This is splenic marginal zone lymphoma. The immunophenotype has no distinctive features but helps to exclude a number of alternative diagnoses. This, with the clinical and cytological features, points to the correct diagnosis. Some plasmacytoid differentiation, as shown in this patient, can be a feature.

EMQ 3

Correct answers I, J, A, H, G

1) This is T-PLL. More often there is expression of CD4 without CD8, but there is expression of both antigens in a quarter to a third of cases [4].
2) This is T lymphoblastic leukaemia/lymphoma (T-ALL). The expression of CD1a and TdT and of cCD3 but not SmCD3 indicates that these are precursor cells.
3) This is ATLL. Opportunistic infections, hypercalcaemia and skin infiltration are all quite common.
4) This is T-LGLL. There is an association with rheumatoid arthritis and with Felty syndrome (splenomegaly and neutropenia associated with rheumatoid arthritis). Loss of expression of CD5, CD7 or both is common. There is also

expression of cytotoxic granule proteins: TIA1, granzyme B and granzyme M.
5) This is Sézary syndrome. The high SCC is attributable to the complexity of the nucleus. Circulating neoplastic cells are not usual in mycosis fungoides, except in the terminal phases of the disease.

EMQ 4

Correct answers J, E, C, D, A

1) This is systemic mastocytosis. Mast cell tryptase staining should be done for confirmation. In systemic mastocytosis, the neoplastic cells show aberrant expression of CD2 and CD25 and sometimes express CD30.
2) This is metastatic carcinoma of the breast. Other markers that might be expressed include cytokeratin and HER2 (CD340). Note that the blood film in secondary myelofibrosis may not be readily distinguishable from primary myelofibrosis.
3) Anaplastic large cell lymphoma is divided into ALK-positive and ALK-negative cases with somewhat different characteristics. This is anaplastic large cell lymphoma, ALK negative. Note that, although of T-lineage, not all cases express CD3.
4) This is classical Hodgkin lymphoma. Note that Reed–Sternberg cells may not be seen in bone marrow infiltrates, even though they are present in lymph node biopsies.
5) This is acute panmyelosis with myelofibrosis. There are immature cells of granulocyte lineage expressing CD117 (myeloperoxidase is usually not expressed). E-cadherin is a marker of the erythroid lineage (more sensitive than glycophorin for the detection of early cells of this lineage) and CD42b of megakaryocyte lineage. Blast cells are increased, as indicated by the expression of CD34.

Answers to FRCPath-Type Questions

Case 1

1) The image of the blood film shows two blast cells and three poorly granulated platelets. The immunophenotyping shows the presence of megakaryoblasts. Acute megakaryoblastic leukaemia associated with t(1;22) (p13.3;q13.1); *RBM15-MKL1* sometimes presents as congenital leukaemia but the normal Hb and platelet count make this diagnosis unlikely. Transient abnormal myelopoiesis (TAM) of Down's syndrome is most likely.

2) The first question we should ask is whether the baby has Down's syndrome.

3) Myeloperoxidase and glycophorin A or E-cadherin could also have been informative, to see if there was any granulocytic or erythroid differentiation, but it is clear that the blast cells are of megakaryocytic lineage.

Trisomy 21 and a *GATA1* mutation were detected, confirming this provisional diagnosis. Despite the name, TAM is correctly regarded as transient leukaemia.

Case 2

1) T-lymphoblastic transformation of chronic myeloid leukaemia.
2) This is a very uncommon event.

The cytospin shows a population of medium to large agranular nucleolated apparently lymphoid cells with a fine chromatin pattern. Interspersed are small lymphoid cells with a mature chromatin pattern. The immunophenotype is of a precursor T-cell neoplasm (T lineage as indicated by cCD3 positivity, precursor as indicated by CD34+) with no other lineage-specific marker. The CD117 is therefore aberrant. CD56 is a promiscuous marker appearing in a range of disorders and CD10 may be expressed in T-ALL. The cytogenetic results are in keeping with the prior diagnosis of CML. The findings therefore indicate a T-lymphoid blast crisis of CML. The small lymphoid cells had a mature T-cell immunophenotype and represent reactive T cells.

The incidence of blast transformation has fallen greatly since the introduction of tyrosine kinase inhibitors. Transformation is most often myeloid or B lymphoblastic. T-lymphoblastic transformation is quite uncommon.

Case 3

1) The most likely diagnosis is meningeal relapse of AML.

The large non-granular cells were gated for analysis (blast gate based on FSC/SSC). The immunophenotype was CD34+, CD117+, CD15+, CD13+, CD33+, HLA-DR+, cCD3– and MPO+. B-lineage and other T-lineage markers were negative. Cytogenetic analysis failed.

The cytospin shows a very cellular CSF, which is grossly abnormal with pleomorphic nucleolated blast cells and myeloid maturation to neutrophils. Some cells show monocytic type morphology but beware of distortion caused by the forces generated by the cytospin preparation. Morphological features such as these are never seen in health.

The differential diagnosis includes a reactive response to bacterial infection or CSF involvement by a myeloid neoplasm. The presence of myeloid precursors is highly suggestive of the latter and, in view of the prior clinical history, this has to be carefully considered. The immunophenotypic analysis identifies a precursor myeloid population. The provisional diagnosis of meningeal relapse of AML is thus confirmed by the immunophenotyping.

It is important to note that MRI imaging often identifies meningeal enhancement in patients with neoplastic meningitis; however, in some patients the imaging is normal. If meningeal disease is still suspected clinically, CSF analysis is still justified.

Case 4

1) The most likely diagnosis is a non-haemopoietic neoplasm.

The marrow aspirate shows sheets of cells with round or ovoid nuclei and minimal cytoplasm. There are a number of bare nuclei. Figure 4.4c shows the disease cell population (red) to be CD45 negative (the black events are normal lymphocytes). It is therefore important to consider that these cells could be non-haemopoietic and notably no lineage-specific marker was identified by flow cytometry. CD117, HLA-DR and CD56 are not lineage specific and can be expressed in non-haemopoietic tumours.

The bone marrow trephine biopsy specimen was heavily infiltrated by intermediate-sized cells with scanty cytoplasm arranged in nests and sheets. Immunohistochemistry showed expression of CAM5.2, AE1/AE3, CD56, chromogranin, synaptophysin and TTF1. There was no expression of CD45, CD3, CD20 or PAX5.

A small cell lung carcinoma was felt to be the most likely diagnosis.

Case 5

1) The most likely diagnosis is acute mono-cytic leukaemia.
2) The lineage is confirmed by the immunophenotyping.

There is a large population of cells of monocytic lineage. These are predominantly promonocytes though small numbers of mature and immature monocytes are also present. A single neutrophil is noted (Figure 4.5a, left), which has virtually agranular cytoplasm. The FSC/SSC characteristics shown in Figure 4.5c and the antigen expression shown in Figure 4.5d demonstrate that the large cells have a predominant CD14+ CD64+ phenotype, confirming their monocytic lineage.

The full immunophenotype was CD34–, CD117–, CD15+, CD13+ (partial), CD33+, HLA-DR+, CD14+, CD64+, cCD3–, CD79a– and MPO+. Other T- and B-lineage markers were negative.

Cytogenetic and molecular genetic analysis showed 46,XY, *NPM1* mutated, *FLT3* wild type.

The diagnosis here is acute monocytic leukaemia. It is absolutely crucial in cases such as this to identify the promonocytes morphologically since they are considered to be blast equivalents. Importantly, the flow cytometry identifies the abnormal cells as being of monocytic lineage but does not show immaturity/phenotypic aberrancy. Monoblasts frequently do not express CD14 so confirmation of immaturity by immunophenotyping is straightforward and the proportion of such cells can easily be quantified. The identification and quantitation of promonocytes, however, relies on careful morphological assessment.

Figures. 4.17a-d illustrate the key morphological features of each phase of maturation of monocytic lineage cells.

(a)

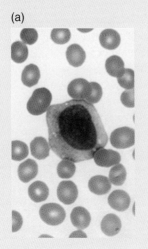

Figure 4.17a Monoblast (×100).

(b)

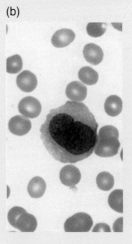

Figure 4.17b Promonocyte (×100).

(c)

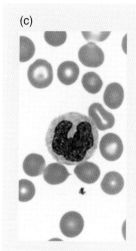

(d)

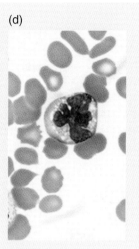

Figure 4.17c   Immature monocyte (×100).   **Figure 4.17d**   Mature monocyte (×100).

Case 6

1) The dominant population shows expression of CD4, CD7, CD33, CD56, CD123 and HLA-DR.
2) Consideration of the morphology and the immunophenotype suggests a diagnosis of blastic plasmacytoid dendritic cell neoplasm.

The presentation with skin lesions and circulating blast cells is important when considering the differential diagnosis. Conditions to consider would be:

- Acute myeloid leukaemia (particularly acute monocytic or monoblastic) with leukaemia cutis
- Blastic plasmacytoid dendritic cell neoplasm

The cells in the film show blastoid morphology with prominent nucleoli and multiple nuclear clefts and lobulation. Note the single dysplastic hypogranular neutrophil. The immunophenotype is unusual. The CD4 and CD7 expression does not reflect T lineage as cCD3 is negative. This is not a monocytic

leukaemia as CD15, CD14 and CD64 are not expressed. No lineage-specific marker is present and cytogenetic analysis was uninformative. However, the phenotype here is typical of blastic plasmacytoid dendritic cell neoplasm. The most characteristic markers are CD4, CD56 and CD123, the latter being positive in most, if not all, cases. Note the partial expression of CD7 and CD56 and the small monocyte population expressing CD14 and CD123 whilst the majority of cells are CD123+, CD14–.

This is a poorly understood condition which often presents with single or multiple skin tumours in parallel with, or shortly followed by, a leukaemic phase. There is no recurring cytogenetic abnormality. The morphology is variable; the cells are usually small to medium size, the nuclei show nucleoli and sometimes clefts as in this case. The cytoplasm is agranular and sometimes contains small vacuoles. In bone marrow aspirates, cells sometimes have cytoplasmic tails. Many cases show dysplastic features in

(continued)

the neutrophil lineage. The condition carries a poor prognosis. There is no consensus on whether AML-type therapy or intensive lymphoma-type therapy provides better outcomes but allogeneic transplantation should be considered in first complete remission in young patients. The condition is uncommon but available evidence suggests meningeal relapse is not uncommon. In patients with skin lesions, it is important to biopsy these

and get cross correlation on diagnosis using immunohistochemistry.

The patient was successfully treated with CODOX M/IVAC chemotherapy. However, two years later he presented with headache. CSF cytology showed abnormal cells similar to those present in blood at diagnosis. Immunophenotyping showed characteristics identical to that at presentation (Figures 4.18a and b).

(a)
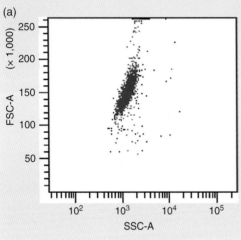
Figure 4.18a

(b)
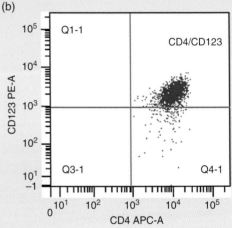
Figure 4.18b

Case 7

1) Acute monoblastic leukaemia.
2) Such striking erythrocyte abnormality as a feature of dyserythropoiesis is quite unusual. Should an underlying inherited condition be suspected?
3) In addition to liver and spleen, gums, skin, lungs, kidneys and CNS.

The film shows a large cell population with typical morphology of monoblasts. Note the large cell size, the ovoid nucleus, prominent nucleoli and copious cytoplasm with fine granules and vacuoles. The monoblasts were easily gated (Figure 4.19a) and in contrast to

Case 5 these cells show expression of CD64 but complete absence of CD14 (Figure 4.19b).

The full phenotype was CD4+, CD13+, CD33+, HLA-DR+, CD64+, CD34−, CD117−, CD14−, cCD3−, CD79a−, CD19− and MPO weak.

Cytogenetic analysis showed 46,XX,del(20)(q11q13).

The diagnosis of acute monoblastic leukaemia is confirmed. We do however need to explain the red cell changes. There are frequent elongated cells, elliptocytes, pencil cells and tear drop poikilocytes. These features appear very extreme to be explained by the dyserythropoiesis that may be seen in acute myeloid leukaemia. However, the patient did in fact have a prior diagnosis of MDS associated with del(20)(q11q13). Prior to this diagnosis being made, she had been considered to have well-compensated hereditary elliptocytosis. However, there have been at least 17 reports of acquired elliptocytosis in patients with a myeloid neoplasm (mainly MDS) associated with del(20q), possible due to deletion of the *EPB41L1* gene at 20q11.23

[5, 6]. One therefore has to consider the possibility that the elliptocytosis was acquired and was the first manifestation of MDS rather than the cytological features being due to the interaction of an inherited and an acquired haematological abnormality.

Acute monoblastic leukaemia has a tendency to affect extramedullary sites; the gingivae, skin, lungs, kidneys and CNS can all be involved either at diagnosis or at relapse.

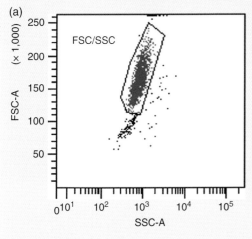

Figure 4.19a

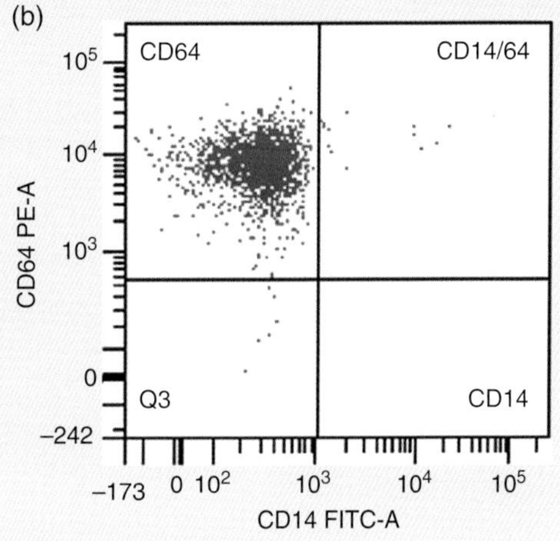

Figure 4.19b

Case 8

1) The most likely diagnosis is therapy-related acute leukaemia, possibly therapy-related acute lymphoblastic leukaemia.
2) The flow cytometry confirms B-ALL and, given the prior therapy and the lineage, rearrangement of *KMT2A* (previously known as *MLL*) could be suspected.

Note the very high WBC. The pleomorphic blast cells show variation in size and nuclear chromatin pattern; some smaller cells show more condensed chromatin. Many larger blasts have nucleoli and multiple nuclear clefts. No granules are visible and there are very few

neutrophils. One could consider the possibility of two populations of cells here (e.g. Richter transformation of CLL). However, the lymphoblasts of ALL can show a size range and variation in chromatin condensation such as is seen here and, given the history, therapy-related ALL could be suspected.

The immunophenotype indicates a precursor B-cell neoplasm that is CD10 negative, namely pro-B-ALL. CD15 expression is aberrant (since MPO is negative). Pro-B-ALL with aberrant myeloid antigen expression, particularly CD15, is often seen in infant B-ALL but can also be seen in sporadic

(continued)

adult B-ALL and in therapy-related B-ALL. Common to all these are translocations involving *KMT2A* at 11q23.3 with a variety of translocation partners.

Cytogenetic studies demonstrated 47,XY,+X, t(11;19)(q23.3;p13.3)[10]. The translocation partner here is *MLLT3* which can be implicated in both myeloid and lymphoid neoplasms. We often assume that a therapy-related neoplasm will be of myeloid lineage. Though this is frequently the case, therapy-related ALL is a real entity and accounts for around 10% of all cases of ALL [7]. The drugs implicated are topoisomerase II inhibitors; the latency period is short at 1 to 3 years, and the prognosis is poor. Allogeneic transplantation in first remission should be considered.

Case 9

1) T-ALL

The findings are of a precursor T-cell neoplasm, cCD3+, CD7+. The unusual finding here is the potential B lineage as suggested by the CD79a expression. In order to confirm B lineage, as recommended by the WHO, a second B-cell marker needs to be expressed. In this case, CD19 was not expressed on the surface or within the cytoplasm of the neoplastic cells so B-lineage specificity and a mixed phenotype leukaemia (MPAL) have not been confirmed. The final diagnosis is T-ALL.

Case 10

1) T prolymphocytic leukaemia
2) Anaplastic large cell lymphoma, ALK-positive

The film shows small lymphoid cells with mature chromatin, nuclear clefts, scanty basophilic cytoplasm and prominent cytoplasmic blebs. There are reactive neutrophils with toxic granulation. The blood film morphology has features that might be in keeping with T-PLL. However, the immunophenotyping, gating on the small lymphoid cells, shows a T-lineage neoplasm, with a minimalistic phenotype, uniform CD26 expression and positivity for CD30. T-PLL normally retains a pan-T immunophenotype and does not express CD30. Furthermore, the genetic studies in this patient show an informative ins(2)t(2;5) (p23;q35q13), a complex variant of the more usual t(2;5)(p23;q35), which indicates a translocation between *ALK* (2p23) and *NPM1* (5q35). This essentially confirms a diagnosis of ALK+ anaplastic large cell lymphoma but, with the morphology, this has to be the small cell variant of this disease. The diagnosis was confirmed on immunohistochemical studies on the bone marrow trephine biopsy and lymph node biopsy specimens. ALK protein staining on the lymph node showed nuclear staining rather than the nuclear plus cytoplasmic staining that is typical of the large cell variant. FISH studies confirmed rearrangement of the *ALK* locus at 2p23.

This is a good example of how clinical, morphological, immunophenotypic and genetic data can be integrated to reach a unified, WHO-recognised diagnosis.

Case 11

1) Hereditary spherocytosis
2) Flow cytometry to show reduced binding of eosin-5-maleimide (EMA)

The history describes an icteric episode in an anaemic patient following an acute gastrointestinal illness. The blood film shows prominent spherocytes, polychromasia and a few acanthocytes. Notably there are no red cell fragments visible and the platelet count is preserved. As the direct Coombs test is negative, an acquired autoimmune haemolytic anaemia, including paroxysmal cold haemoglobinuria, is unlikely. Flow cytometry studies for red cell EMA binding were requested and are shown in Figure 4.20.

The patient/control EMA binding ratio was abnormal at 0.53 (NR >0.8). This finding together with the blood film morphology and the presenting history are in keeping with an acute haemolytic episode triggered by a gastrointestinal illness in a patient with hereditary spherocytosis.

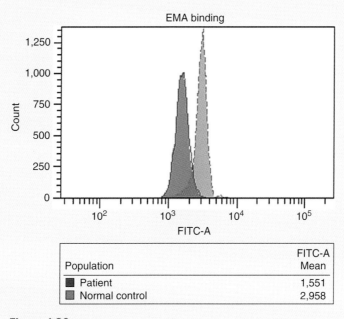

Population	FITC-A Mean
■ Patient	1,551
■ Normal control	2,958

Figure 4.20

Case 12

1) An acquired haemolytic anaemia should be suspected and, given the thrombocytopenia, paroxysmal nocturnal haemoglobinuria (PNH) needs to be considered.
2) Inspection of the urine and microscopy is needed to confirm the 'haematuria'. Flow cytometric analysis of erythrocytes, neutrophils and monocytes to confirm a diagnosis of PNH is indicated.

It is often important in medicine to confirm reported observations or laboratory findings that are key to a differential diagnosis. If this is not done, the diagnostic pathway can be

(continued)

seriously disrupted. It is therefore important to carefully assess patients such as this. The haematology trainee did exactly this and his observation of the urine in the bladder irrigation catheter bag was key to the diagnosis. Rather than noting the bright red/pink urine of frank haematuria he noted a rather dark discoloured urine resembling Coca Cola. This urine finding is typical of haemoglobinuria and is a key finding in patients with intravascular haemolysis. The differential diagnosis is now distinctly changed, and investigations take on an entirely new pathway.

Laboratory features are certainly in keeping with a haemolytic anaemia with raised bilirubin, LDH and AST (released from lysed red cells). However, the reticulocytosis is mild and there is also thrombocytopenia; these two features need to be explained. The blood film shows mild non-specific red cell changes with anisopoikilocytosis but notably no fragments, ghost cells or agglutinates (considering possible diagnoses of microangiopathic haemolytic anaemia, paroxysmal cold haemoglobinuria, glucose-6 phosphate dehydrogenase deficiency and cold autoimmune haemolytic anaemia respectively). The relative low reticulocyte count and thrombocytopenia might indicate a concurrent bone marrow hypoplasia and bone marrow trephine biopsy did show reduced cellularity at 25%, without erythroid expansion and

with reduced numbers of megakaryocytes. No abnormal infiltrate was identified.

The diagnosis of PNH thus needs to be considered. PNH is a haemopoietic stem cell disorder characterised by the triad of intravascular haemolysis, bone marrow failure/hypoplasia and thrombosis. Typically, these three features do not all present at the same time point. The pathogenesis appears to relate to mutations in the *PIGA* gene, which encodes a glycosylphosphatidyl inositol (GPI) anchor of normal blood cell membranes. Loss of this anchor raft leads to a loss of surface antigens and some of these have important roles, notably in protection of cells from inappropriate complement activation and from thrombosis. A flow cytometric assessment of granulocyte CD24 versus FLAER and CD66 binding is shown for this patient in Figures 4.21a and b. CD24 and CD66 are both GPI-anchored proteins and the fluorochrome-labelled inactivated bacterial haemolysin derivative, FLAER, binds directly to the GPI anchor.

These studies demonstrate a large population of neutrophils showing complete loss of these antigens and FLAER binding indicating a type III PNH clone at 90% of events. The large clone size explains the intravascular haemolysis and also presents a significant thrombotic risk for the patient. He was subsequently anticoagulated with warfarin and commenced eculizumab therapy.

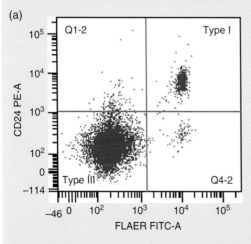

(a)

Figure 4.21a

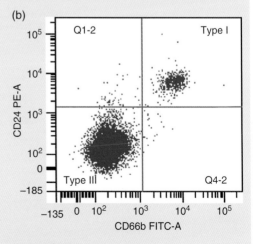

(b)

Figure 4.21b

Case 13

1) The CLL score is 1/5.
2) This is a non-Hodgkin lymphoma, most likely splenic marginal zone lymphoma.
3) The patient does not currently need any treatment.

This patient has an incidental finding of a moderate peripheral blood lymphocytosis. The blood film shows lymphocytes with a condensed chromatin pattern, some nuclear indentations and cytoplasmic tufts.

The immunophenotype is of a mature clonal CD5+ B-cell lymphoproliferative disorder with a CLL score of only 1/5 (1 point for CD5+) [8] making this diagnosis unlikely. Other characteristics suggesting that this is not CLL are the strong CD20 expression (note the co-expression of bright CD20 and CD5 in Figure 4.13d) and negativity for CD200 and LEF1. Failure to express cyclin D1 and SOX11 excludes mantle cell lymphoma leaving a favoured diagnosis of splenic marginal zone lymphoma. The patient does not currently require treatment as there are no cytopenias and the splenomegaly is asymptomatic.

Case 14

1) AML and acute undifferentiated leukaemia
2) Acute undifferentiated leukaemia (AUL)

This case needs to be worked through carefully if we are to make a correct diagnosis. The patient presented with a short history, rib and chest wall pain and a mild pancytopenia. The marrow shows a marked excess of medium to large ovoid blast cells with prominent multiple nucleoli and without discernible granules. The neutrophils show marked hypogranularity.

The blasts show no lineage-specific marker but do express some myeloid antigens (CD13, CD33) together with CD34, HLA-DR, CD7 and TdT. The metaphase cytogenetic profile is normal and no *BCR-ABL1* fusion transcript, *FLT3* ITD or *NPM1* mutation was identified.

In order to try and refine the diagnosis further, a lymph node biopsy was taken. This showed foci of blastoid cells amongst normal CD4+ and CD8+ T cells: the large cells expressed strong CD7, weak CD2, CD3 and CD5 and absence of CD4 and CD8. CD10, CD20, CD30, CD56, CD57, PAX5 and ALK1 were not expressed. The bone marrow trephine biopsy also highlighted these cells, showing expression of CD34, TdT, CD7 and CD5 but provided no additional information.

According to the 2016 WHO classification [1], this is acute undifferentiated leukaemia but in view of the hypogranular neutrophils, one would be tempted to think that it is actually myeloid. AUL is a poorly understood entity, which probably arises from a bone marrow stem cell. The prognosis is generally poor and there is no consensus on the optimal approach to therapy (AML or ALL type treatment). This patient did unfortunately prove refractory to both AML and ALL type induction chemotherapy and treatment was purely supportive thereafter.

Case 15

1) T-cell large granular lymphocytic leukaemia (LGL leukaemia)
2) T-cell receptor (*TRDC*) analysis to demonstrate clonality and molecular analysis to demonstrate any mutation relevant to diagnosis and possibly to management.

This patient has a significant degree of anaemia and neutropenia associated with peripheral blood T-cell excess. The blood film shows prominent mature granulated lymphocytes and these have a CD8+ phenotype. Such populations can be seen as a reactive phenomenon to other stimuli, in particular, viral infection, when they often express HLA-DR. The multiple antigen loss in this case, CD7, CD5 and CD26, suggests a clonal LGL population. This, however, must be confirmed particularly if we believe these cells are implicated in the cytopenias in which case specific therapy will be indicated. The bone marrow aspirate and trephine biopsy showed a similar CD8+ T-cell infiltrate. Cellularity was 15–20%, with preserved myeloid precursors but little maturation to neutrophils. There were no significant dysplastic features.

In view of these findings, the patient's peripheral blood lymphocytes underwent next generation sequencing studies of *STAT3* and *STAT5B* genes. There was no mutation of *STAT5B* but *STAT3* (mutated in about a third of cases) showed an exon 21 mutation, p.Y640F C.1919A>T.

This finding is important in a number of respects. Firstly, it confirms that the diagnosis here is a clonal LGL leukaemia and not a reactive phenomenon. It is therefore likely that this T-cell population is implicated in the cytopenias, notably not by anatomical occupation of the bone marrow space but by cytokine-mediated mechanisms within the bone marrow milieu, and that specific directed treatment is indicated. A number of drugs have been advocated for treating this condition, those most favoured being ciclosporin, cyclophosphamide and methotrexate. Recent reports have investigated the use of gene sequencing as a means of guiding initial therapy. One such study reports frequent responses to methotrexate used first line in *STAT3* Y640F mutated T LGL leukaemia [9]. This patient has commenced treatment with methotrexate and both the anaemia and neutropenia have resolved.

Case 16

1) Prominent type I and II haematogones. No blast population.
2) The preservation of normal cell lines, typical immunophenotypes of type I and II haematogones, the size of the haematogone population and the age of the patient. Haematogones are often prominent in paediatric bone marrow specimens particularly in young children and infants. They are often prominent in reactive marrows and are not normally associated with primary bone marrow disease.

This child underwent a bone marrow examination in order to exclude an acute leukaemia. The aspirate did show areas of prominent lymphoid cells showing varying degrees of morphological maturity and importantly the erythroid, myeloid and megakaryocyte lineages were preserved. On first inspection of the immunophenotyping, there might be concern regarding a population of cells with the phenotype of common ALL. It is very important to examine the scatter plots in this situation. The CD45 versus SSC plot indicates there are 2 populations with reduced CD45 expression (labelled I and II in Figure 4.16c).

The two populations have different phenotypes as illustrated in Figures 4.16d, 4.16e and 4.16f. These populations represent type I and type II haematogones. The type I cells are CD79a+, CD19^{weak}, CD10^{strong}, TdT+, CD20− and CD34+ (not shown) whilst the type II cells show a more mature CD79a+, CD19+, CD10+, TdT− and CD20^{variable} phenotype. No discrete blast population was identified. The child made an uneventful recovery from the febrile episode.

References

1 Swerdlow SH, Campo E, Harris NL, Jaffe ES, Pileri S, Stein H and Thiele J (eds) (2017) *WHO Classification of Tumours of Haematopoietic and Lymphoid Tissues*, revised 4th edn. IARC Press, Lyon.

2 Park BG, Chi HS, Jang S, Park CJ, Kim DY, Lee JH *et al.* (2013) Association of cup-like nuclei in blasts with *FLT3* and *NPM1* mutations. *Ann Hematol*, **92**, 451–457.

3 McKay P, Leach M, Jackson B, Robinson S and Rule S (2018) A British Society for Haematology good practice paper on the diagnosis and investigation of patients with mantle cell lymphoma. *Br J Haematol*, **182**, 63–70.

4 Chen X and Cherian S (2013) Immunophenotypic characterization of T-cell prolymphocytic leukemia. *Am J Clin Pathol*, **140**, 727–735.

5 Boutault R and Eveillard M (2016) Acquired elliptocytosis in the setting of a refractory anemia with excess blasts and del(20q). *Blood*, **127**, 2646–2646.

6 Kjelland J D, Dwyre DM and Jonas BA (2017) Acquired elliptocytosis as a manifestation of myelodysplastic syndrome with ring sideroblasts and multilineage dysplasia. *Case Reports in Hematology*, **2017**: 3625946.

7 Aldoss I, Stiller T, Tsai NC, Song JY, Cao T, Bandara NA *et al.* (2018) Therapy-related acute lymphoblastic leukaemia has distinct clinical and cytogenetic features compared to *de novo* acute lymphoblastic leukaemia but outcomes are comparable in transplanted patients. *Haematologica*, **103**, 1662–1668.

8 Matutes E, Owusu-Ankomah K, Morilla R, Garcia-Marco J, Houlihan A, Que TH and Catovsky D (1994) The immunological profile of B-cell disorders and proposal of a scoring system for the diagnosis of CLL. *Leukemia*, **8**, 1640–1645.

9 Loughran TP, Zickl L, Olson TL, Wang V, Zhang D, Rajala HL *et al.* (2015). Immunosuppressive therapy of LGL leukemia: prospective multicenter phase II study by the Eastern Cooperative Oncology Group (E5998). *Leukemia*, **29**, 886−894.

Further Reading

Leach M, Drummond M, Doig A, McKay P, Jackson R and Bain BJ (2015) Practical Flow Cytometry in Haematology: 100 worked examples, Wiley-Blackwell, Oxford.

British Society for Haematology https://b-s-h.org.uk/education/bsh-education-resources/multiple-choice-questions/ https://b-s-h.org.uk/education/bsh-education-resources/extended-matching-questions/

Examination advice from the Royal College of Pathologists https://www.rcpath.org/trainees/examinations/examinations-by-specialty/haematology.html (Sample MCQs, EMQs and sample part 2 questions are provided.)

Index

Note: Page numbers in *italic* refer to figures, those in **bold** refer to tables.

Immunophenotyping for Haematologists: Principles and Practice, First Edition. Barbara J. Bain and Mike Leach.
© 2021 John Wiley & Sons Ltd. Published 2021 by John Wiley & Sons Ltd.